The Complete Idiot's Re

Knowledge is power, so we tracked down these great, consumer-oriented government health Websites. Many of these sites have won awards, they can handle a large volume of inquiries, and they are kept up to date.

Agency for Health Care Policy and Research: www.ahcpr.gov/consumer
Clinical guidelines written for consumers
choosing health plans.

Centers for Disease Control and Prevention: www.cdc.gov
Infectious diseases, immunization, physical
activity, tobacco, sexually transmitted diseases.

Centers for Disease Control and Prevention Travel Site www.cdc.gov/travel/

Consumer Information Center: www.pueblo.gsa.gov
The big file box of dozens of health topics.

Consumer Product Safety Comm.: www.cpsc.gov
Recalls—have you been hurt by something
you bought?

Department of Agriculture Center for Nutrition Policy and Promotion: http://usda.gov/fcs/cnpp.htm
Food and nutrition.

Environmental Protection Agency: www.epa.gov
Environment and human health risk.

Food and Drug Administration: www.fda.gov
What you eat, prescription drugs, cosmetics,
and medical devices.

Health Care Financing Administration: www.hcfa.gov
Medicare and Medicaid info.

Healthfinders: www.healthfinder.gov
Thousands of consumer and human services
topics, support groups, and more.

National AIDS Clearinghouse Centers for Disease Control: www.cdcnac.org
AIDS/HIV info source.

continues

alpha
books

continued

National Center for Alcohol and Drug Information:
Just what it says.

www.health.org

National Cancer Institute:
The latest cancer info.

http://cancernet.nci.nih.gov

National Heart, Lung and Blood Institute

www.nhlbi.nih.gov/nhlbi.htm

National Institute of Diabetes and Digestive and Kidney Diseases:
Everything you wanted to know about these subjects.

www.niddk.nih.gov

National Institute of Health:
The Nation's premier biomedical research center.

www.nih.gov

National Institute of Mental Health:
Here's the science.

www.nimh.nih.gov

National Library of Medicine:
Research-oriented reference site— the grandaddy of medical libraries.

www.nlm.nih.gov

National Mental Health Knowledge Exchange Network, Substance Abuse and Mental Health Services Administration:
Here's the research.

www.mentalhealth.org

NIH Office of Alternative Medicine:
The government's research office for new and old remedies.

http://altmed.od.nih.gov/oam

U.S. Administration on Aging:
Aging and the elderly.

www.aoa.dhhs.gov

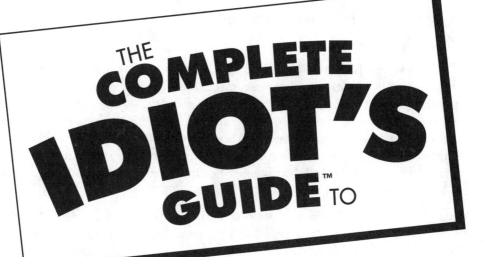

THE COMPLETE IDIOT'S GUIDE™ TO

Managed Health Care

by Sophie M. Korczyk, Ph.D.
and Hazel A. Witte, Esq.

alpha books

A Division of Macmillan General Reference
A Simon and Schuster Macmillan Company
1633 Broadway, New York NY 10019-6785

We dedicate this book to our children.

©1998 Alpha Books

Macmillan Publishing books may be purchased for business or sales promotional use. For information please write: Special Markets Department, Macmillan Publishing USA, 1633 Broadway, New York, NY 10019.

THE COMPLETE IDIOT'S GUIDE name and design are trademarks of Macmillan, Inc.

International Standard Book Number: 0-02-861165-4
Library of Congress Catalog Card Number: 97-80951

00 99 98   4 3 2 1

Interpretation of the printing code: the rightmost number of the first series of numbers is the year of the book's printing; the rightmost number of the second series of numbers is the number of the book's printing. For example, a printing code of 98-1 shows that the first printing occurred in 1998.

Printed in the United States of America

Alpha Development Team
Brand Manager
Kathy Nebenhaus

Director of Editorial Services
Brian Phair

Executive Editor
Gary M. Krebs

Managing Editor
Bob Shuman

Senior Editor
Nancy Mikhail

Development Editors
Jennifer Perillo, Amy Zavatto

Production Team
Development Editor
Sharron Wood

Production Editor
Mark Enochs

Editorial Assistant
Maureen Horn

Cartoonist
Judd Winick

Book Designer
Glenn Larsen

Cover Designer
Michael Freeland

Indexers
Chris Barrick, Becky Hornyak

Production Team
Tricia Flodder, Mary Hunt, Lisa Stumpf, Megan Wade

Contents at a Glance

Contents

9 Beyond the Big City: Managed Care in Rural Areas   95

10 Medicaid   105

Foreword

When pollsters or academic researchers ask us how we regard our health plans, the American public rapidly divides into two camps. People who have been with the same health plan for many years generally are quite satisfied. They trust their doctors and they know how to get the care they want—with a minimum of hassle. But people who are just starting out with a new medical-insurance plan—particularly people entering the world of managed care for the first time—are much more likely to be frustrated and bewildered. They find themselves in an unfamiliar system full of rules and obstacles that emerge without warning. For those consumers, trying to get good care is a bit like trying to drive through Barcelona at night without a map.

Until now, there hasn't been any quick way to pick up the expertise needed to make sense of managed care. Friends and neighbors might pass along the occasional tip. Doctors and nurses, if asked, might try to help patients sort their way through a particularly baffling part of the health plan maze. But many people delivering medical care have been struggling just as much as their patients to understand the new insurance rules. In such an environment, it can take years for consumers to master the system.

Fortunately, Sophie Korczyk and Hazel Witte have stepped forward to fill that void. Their new book is a timely, wide-ranging, and refreshingly clear explanation of the managed care environment. At every step of the way, Sophie and Hazel champion the consumer's point of view. Rather than get bogged down in political theories or the intricacies of health care finance, the authors focus on what each health plan member needs to know most: how to make the right medical choices in our day-to-day lives.

Not only is this a very pragmatic book, it is fundamentally an optimist's book as well. Sophie and Hazel start by explaining how different health plans work, and how to choose the right one for you and your family. They progress through all the choices that come next: how to pick a primary care doctor; how to get referrals to specialists; how to get good care of a chronic illness, and how to become a "special" patient in a system that doesn't always make allowances for the individual. In each chapter, the authors acknowledge flaws with current-day managed care. But they believe that with the right skills and tactics, it is possible for consumers to get much better results. As they tell us in Chapter 3, "The Informed Consumer Gets the Best Health Care."

For many consumers, health care choices don't command attention as long as we are healthy. But a small amount of preparation can be a literal lifesaver if illness strikes. At the very least, that means learning the rules of managed care. For too long, both medicine and health insurance have been shrouded with jargon and obscure technical knowledge, until the average layperson has been at the mercy of the experts. Things don't need to be that way.

The rise of managed care has occurred so quickly and quietly that most people don't fully fathom its importance. A better understanding of managed care's promises and pitfalls should be high on almost every consumer's priority list. Fortunately, many aspects of patient care and insurance coverage can be explained clearly and directly, so that we can make the choices we want. The explanations and common-sense advice in this book are an important step forward in that process.

George Anders

George Anders is the author of *Health Against Wealth* (Houghton Mifflin, 1996), one of the first in-depth examinations of the HMO industry. That book was called a must-read by the *Journal of the American Medical Association* and was hailed by the *Washington Post* as "a chilling look at the revolutionary changes taking place in the medical marketplace." Mr. Anders' articles on business and health issues have appeared in *Harvard Business Review*, the *Chicago Tribune*, *Stanford* magazine, and other national publications. His first book, *Merchants of Debt* (Basic Books, 1992), was acclaimed by the *New York Times* as a "refreshing and important" account of Wall Street intrigue. He lives in the the San Francisco Bay Area with his wife and son.

Introduction

One health guru said, in all seriousness, that anybody who thinks they understand their health insurance doesn't understand the problem.

How could that be? Everyone needs to go to the doctor, even if only on rare occasions.

But he was right. You could get dizzy just trying to get through voice mail to ask your plan a question.

We wanted to write something that could explain how a perplexing, sometimes mystifying system works. Then, inspiration! Why don't we use the same approach that works with Windows 95, Excel, or almost anything else explained in the *Idiots* series: describe a system, explain how it works, and explain how to troubleshoot it.

That's our goal. Health care is a big-ticket item. You pay a lot for it, whether it comes out of your paycheck or your bank account. In fact, the reason managed health care has spread like wildfire in the '90s is the promise to keep cost down by limiting choices.

But capping the cost doesn't do justice to what has happened to the health care system. Health care has morphed into an entirely new form: "Come to our plan! We've got rules and more rules, three types of medical directors, and a database the size of Texas."

Even as we wrote this book, we lived through many of the problems that surface when you use health care. We've changed plans, used specialists, worked through billing problems, sent kids to college, used preventive care, and delved into Medicare questions for our parents.

We know, personally and professionally, that your life depends on the choices you make—and sometimes you don't even know you have choices. We hope the ideas and information put forth in this book give you the support you need to get the health care you want, need, and deserve.

What You'll Learn in This Book

This book is divided into five parts. Five easy pieces, to help you make sense of your managed care plan—and everyone else's, too. We start you with the easy stuff, and before you know it, you're ready to make decisions about brain surgery. Yes, really!

In Part 1, "Getting Your Bearings," we lay it all out for you. Who are the managed health care players? What game are they playing? And, most importantly, what are the rules, how do you find them out, and how do you play to win?

Part 2, "Choosing (and Paying for) Your Coverage," is about getting health care coverage. There are different paths for different folks, depending on whether you work or have retired, whether you work for IBM or for yourself, where you live, and whether you can get Uncle Sam to contribute. We also tell you how to find out if your managed care plan has the right seal of approval (or, indeed, any at all).

Part 3, "Using Your Plan," is about using your managed care plan day to day. It's about primary care, preventive care, and the occasional emergency, as well as the different ways men and women think about health care.

In Part 4, "Above and Beyond: When You Need Special Care," we bring you into the world of specialist care. We start with maternity care (doesn't everyone?), then cover chronic conditions, major illnesses and injuries, treatments the medical field is only learning about, mental health and substance abuse treatment, and getting your managed care plan to pay when you're out of town. Then, just in case you think we're getting too serious, we end with the little extras—some of them not so little—that your managed care plan may offer to attract you and keep you healthy and happy.

Part 5, "Your Right to the Right Care," is about who's in your corner when you really need someone. We go over what they know about you: your medical records. We also tell you what you need to know about them. We tell you how to convince your plan to see it your way, whether in an appeal, arbitration, court, or complaint to state or federal regulators.

Bonus Beacons

In addition to all the explanations and checklists, this book contains other types of information to make it even easier for you to understand your health care plan.

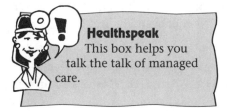

Healthspeak
This box helps you talk the talk of managed care.

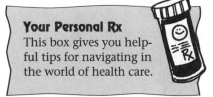

Your Personal Rx
This box gives you helpful tips for navigating in the world of health care.

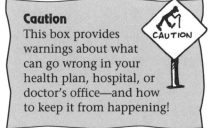

Caution
This box provides warnings about what can go wrong in your health plan, hospital, or doctor's office—and how to keep it from happening!

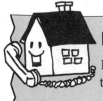

House Call
Look here for expert advice, true stories, and other health care information.

Acknowledgments

We would like to thank everyone who gave their time and thoughts to this project, including doctors, lawyers, business executives, managed care plan officials, and just plain patients. It was gratifying to have so many people respond so quickly and thoroughly to our inquiries. "Make sure you put this in" or "You have to tell people what to do when this happens" took the place of a wave goodbye at the school bus stop, professional meetings, conferences, and family reunions.

We would also like to thank our editorial manager, Robert Shuman; our editor, Sharron Wood, for a marvelously easy working relationship; and our agent Tim Seldes.

A special thanks to our husbands, whose patience, encouragement, and humor were ever present and always appreciated, and our children, who understood so graciously when Mom was busy.

Special Thanks to the Technical Reviewer

The *Complete Idiot's Guide to Managed Health Care* was reviewed by an expert who checked the technical accuracy of what you learned in this book and provided invaluable insight.

William S. Custer, Ph.D., has authored numerous articles and studies on the health care delivery system, heath insurance, retirement income security, and employee benefits. He is currently on the faculty of the Department of Risk Management and Insurance at Georgia State University.

Dr. Custer earned a B.S. in Economics at the University of Minnesota and received his Ph.D. in Economics from the University of Illinois at Urbana. Dr. Custer and his wife, Wendy Nelson, have three children.

Part 1
Getting Your Bearings

So you need to choose a health plan—or understand the one someone (your spouse, maybe your employer) has chosen for you.

Where do you start? What questions do you ask? What do all those colorful brochures with pictures of friendly doctors and cute babies mean to you? And, most importantly, which plan do you want on your side when that cute baby—or you—won't stop crying?

Let's start by getting oriented in the world of managed care, lining up the players and their roles, and figuring out some of the rules of the game.

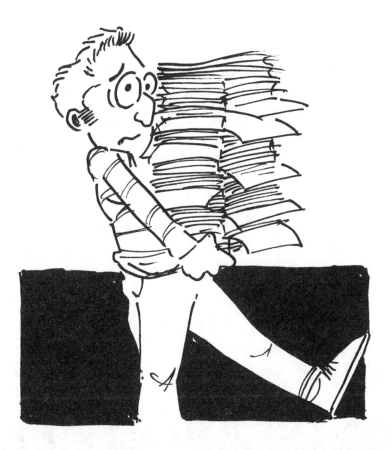

Dear Reader,

Once upon a time, when you got sick, it was just you, your doctor, and a few basic rules. Now it's a cast of hundreds, their voice mail, and a list of rules as long as your arm…in very small type.

This new health care system is called managed care. And we have news for you—it's *you* who are being managed!

We can't bring you chicken soup when you get sick, but we have brought you something better: this book. It is for anyone who belongs to a managed care plan, considers joining one, or has a loved one in one. That covers just about everyone we know. That's why we wrote it.

This book will make staying well, getting the care you need when you are sick, and getting well easier. And it could even save your life!

We've talked to patients, doctors, nurses, employers, and managed care executives. We've talked to lawyers, government workers, insurance agents, and medical researchers. And we've shared with you our own personal and professional experiences in the health care maze. Most of what is in this book is not written down in any one place—and some of it's not written down *anywhere*!

You can read this book straight through and get prepared for anything that might arise. Or you can readily find the information you need to cope with a crisis and deal with your health plan with confidence. We have checklists, question lists, special tips, and a wide array of references on just about any problem you might face. Our goal is to put *you* in the driver's seat.

You *can* survive—even thrive!—in the world of managed care. Let us show you how.

Sophie M. Korczyk

Hazel Witte

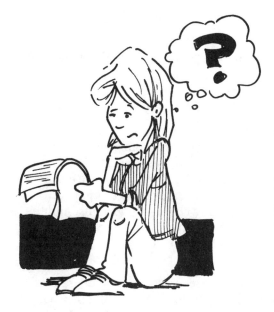

What Managed Care Means to You

"My husband was in terrible pain—just like the kidney stone attack two years ago. It scared me to death, so I ran to the emergency room. Six weeks later, I got a bill for $650.00. My health plan wouldn't pay for the ER because they said I should have called first!" *47-year-old set designer, mother of two.*

"If I have one more patient ask me to fax their referral to a specialist, I'm going to rip out the fax. Would they ask their managers to spend their day faxing?" *Pediatric nurse, 25 years experience.*

These are the sounds of managed health care.

We all learned how to use health care in our childhood. We learned when to call the doctor, what to tell him, and how to act during an appointment. With a good coloring book and favorite soup, bed rest wasn't such a bad deal. We probably went to the same doctor throughout childhood, and figured that the health care universe began and ended there, with a possible visit to the hospital.

Most of us move on to adult life using the same rituals we learned in childhood. But the cold, cruel blast of skyrocketing costs changed that world. *Health care coverage* is probably the most valuable benefit you get from your employer besides your paycheck, and if you buy health care coverage on your own, you can barely catch your breath between premium increases.

> **Healthspeak**
> *Health care coverage* includes insurance policies and memberships in other types of health plans such as health maintenance organizations (HMOs).

In a desperate attempt to keep costs from rising beyond reach, employers and individual buyers are choosing managed care companies for their health care coverage—companies that advertise with an unlimited supply of smiling faces and athletically gifted grandparents. And the names in health care have changed. Your doctor is now a "provider" and part of a "plan" or "network." The patient is now a "member" and receives "services."

This new world order may seem too large and dense to comfortably deal with you, the person now sitting in the doctor's office with one zinger of a sinus infection. So how much do you really need to know about this system? Do you need to know the circuitry intimately, or, like using your television, do you need to know just enough to change the channels? In short, you need to know more than how to work the remote, but you don't need to study electromagnetic theory. This chapter gives you the basics to understanding your managed health care system.

The "Managed" in Managed Care

The best way to begin understanding managed care is to understand what it's not. Modern managed care began as an attempt to reform the traditional or *fee-for-service* method of charging for care. Under this traditional system, doctors and hospitals made more money the more they did, but patients were not always better off. Some patients got care they did not need, while others missed out on necessary care.

> **Healthspeak**
> Under a *fee-for-service* system, a physician, hospital, or other health care provider bills for each service rendered, with no limits or oversight of the treatment decisions. While the terms "indemnity" and "fee-for-service" are not exactly the same thing, they are often used interchangeably. Pure fee-for-service systems have gone the way of the Model T.

Managed care organizations differ quite a bit from each other, but the following are characteristics common to all managed care plans:

➤ They actively supervise the financing of medical care delivered to members. They try to get the biggest bang for their buck by purchasing or writing special contracts with hospitals, physician practices, and other medical organizations.

➤ All managed care organizations actively manage what is called the "delivery system"—who gives care, where they give it, and how many different types of doctors give care in their systems. Delivery systems also include hospitals, therapists, pharmacists, nurses, and others. Some companies manage more actively than others.

➤ Managed care makes primary care physicians the center of care (see Chapter 11 for more on this).

➤ Managed care organizations limit medical services to control costs. How do they do it? They scrutinize doctors' treatment decisions; they put limits on prescription drugs; and they put up hurdles to costly or exceptional treatments. They also negotiate special prices with health care providers.

Any managed care plan limits your choices, providing a list of doctors you choose from, the list of medicines for your doctor to choose, and the list of labs where your tests can be done. But the degree to which your choices are limited depends on the type and quality of your plan. A managed care plan can be a buyer of bulk services—a cost cutter—with less interest in coordinating services. Or it can try to keep costs down by coordinating patient care, educating patients, and keeping an eye out for unnecessary care.

The Alphabet Soup: HMOs, PPOs, POS, and the Rest

Can you do it? Do you know the name of your managed care plan and if it is an HMO, PPO, or some other creature?

Don't hang your head. You might be surprised by the number of people who show up at their doctor's office without a clue, knowing only that they signed up for health care benefits at work. Once upon a time, you could just say "Oh, I have Blue Cross, but the card is at home (maybe spinning in the dryer). I'll get you the number later."

Caution
Unmanaged care is rare. Even in the most traditional plans, you are typically required to get prior approval for hospital stays and surgeries, and get second opinions before the doctor can perform surgery.

Your Personal Rx
You can always expand your choices by not choosing the plan's way, but it will cost you. If you choose not to follow your managed health care plan's rules, you will pay for your medical care out-of-pocket.

Your Personal Rx
Knowing the type of plan you have will give you an idea of what to expect from your plan, what services are covered by your plan, and what it expects from you as a member. It will also tell you to whom you complain (see Chapters 23 and 25). Health plans can also vary a great deal from place to place and from year to year. Make sure to read any updated materials your plan sends to you.

Cost and choice trade-offs in health care plans.

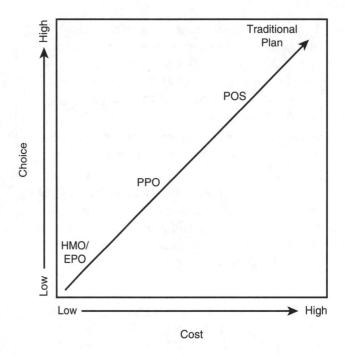

That approach is history. There are many different types of managed care plans, and sometimes the same company offers different types of managed care plans to your employer. Take a few minutes to familiarize yourself with them. For a list of services that each may offer, see Chapter 5.

Health Maintenance Organizations (HMOs)

You walk into the travel agency and pay for your cruise. Ah, what a relief. No extra charges, no add-ons. Everything you want is included in the price, and a pretty good price at that. But you've got to stay on the boat. If you want to visit the island, or try another boat, you are totally on your own. That could be a budget buster.

Health maintenance organizations (HMOs), like the cruise, provide one-stop shopping. You pay for your care ahead of time when you (and/or your employer) pay your health coverage premium. In these arrangements, many doctors are on salary, or belong to a group that services only one HMO, and see only HMO members and only at specific locations.

There are several types of HMOs. (Some folks say, "If you've seen one HMO, you've seen one HMO.") Often, you will see your doctor, get your lab tests and X-rays, have your prescriptions filled, and order your glasses or contact lenses all in one location. These are called *staff model HMOs*.

Think of your local school system. Everyone from the principal to the janitor is in the same building. Some specialists, like speech therapists, are on call at several schools, but all work for the same system.

House Call

When you join an HMO, you are joining a plan, not a doctor's practice. If your doctor leaves the plan, your health care must continue with another HMO doctor. If you want to follow your doctor, you have to pay out-of-pocket or join a new plan.

The focus of your care is the primary care doctor, usually a family practitioner, internist, or pediatrician. They are sometimes known as *gatekeepers*, because they act as sentries for the HMO when services beyond primary are considered. These include referrals to specialists and further diagnostic tests (there's more on this in Chapter 11).

The staff model HMO also employs specialists (or contracts with outside specialists in certain cases). Generally, that specialist is at the same location as your doctor, but may be located at another of the HMO's sites in your community. Your medical records are also kept in a central location, accessible to every doctor who sees you.

Healthspeak
A *gatekeeper* is typically a primary care doctor. All care other than that of the primary care physician or true emergencies must be approved by the patient's primary care physician. This is the cornerstone of care in HMOs and many other types of plans.

An *independent practice association (IPA)* is a physically less restrictive version of an HMO than a staff model. All doctors, both primary and specialists, see patients/plan members in their own offices. They can also have patients from other medical plans. You sometimes have more specialists to choose from in an IPA than in a staff model HMO because they can see members of other plans, giving them a larger patient and income base.

Why would that be important? You may have a larger group of specialists servicing your HMO. Or if you are thinking of changing plans (or your employer thinks of it for you), you won't necessarily have to leave your family doctor. But if you value the one-stop shopping of a staff model HMO, you won't find it in an IPA model HMO.

An *exclusive provider organization (EPO)* has some characteristics of an HMO and some of a PPO. EPOs use primary care doctors as gatekeepers and do not pay for care outside the EPO. In many states they are regulated under state insurance statutes.

Healthspeak
Capitation is a fixed prepayment to a doctor or hospital to deliver medical services to a certain group, such as all the members of a particular health plan.

You may hear about other types of HMOs besides the ones listed above, such as group practice, network, and direct contract. The major differences among these types is how the managed care companies relate to the doctors who treat their members. This is the business side of managed care—where decisions and agreements are reached on what the doctors and plans' obligations are to each other. This includes patient access and referrals and what payment arrangements they will use to pay participating doctors.

Sometimes doctors, mostly primary care doctors, agree to accept members of a plan for a certain price per member and no more, no matter how much they use the doctor. This is called *capitation* because the doctor is paid a specific amount per head or per person for all services within a certain amount of time. For instance, your doctor may receive $20.00 per month for you, whether you see him five times that month or once.

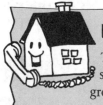

House Call

There are many different ways your doctors can be paid. These compensation arrangements can be very complex. In fact, a whole industry has grown up around physician contracting.

What Is the "Maintenance" in HMOs?

HMOs typically cover preventive care, such as check-ups, health screens, and immunizations. Preventive care is one of their big selling points; they reel in members by promising to keep you healthy and catch any problems before they start (see Chapter 12 for more on preventive care).

HMOs maintain not only your health but also control the quality of your health care. Almost all care must be preapproved, and referrals must usually go through a primary care/gatekeeper doctor. HMOs have made their money and their reputations by reviewing the necessity of medical care, and that review is the cornerstone of their operations. Review of medical care before it happens means that the HMOs can decide about the cost and appropriateness of medical care before taking on any charges. Good HMOs have the opportunity to weed out bad practices before inappropriate treatment is started. Bad HMOs limit care that really is necessary or give you care that is inappropriate.

Preferred Provider Organizations (PPOs)

A *preferred provider organization (PPO)* is a health plan in which a member's health care is largely or completely paid for if they use the doctors and hospitals in the group or network with whom the plan has a contract. If you go out of the network for the doctors or hospitals, it will cost you more (sometimes much more).

How does it work? Employer plans or insurance carriers contract to buy health services from a selected group of doctors, hospitals, and other facilities like laboratories and radiology centers. The doctors and hospitals agree to accept a discounted fee for PPO members. They also agree to some sort of review by the plan of their treatment decisions, including referrals.

Your Personal Rx
A PPO gives you more flexibility than an HMO when picking a doctor, particularly a specialist, but requires you pay part of the fee if you use a doctor outside the network.

Point of Service Plans (POS)

For those who really can't make a commitment (you know who you are), a *point of service plan (POS)* may be the best choice. This type of plan lets you decide—literally at the point of service—which provider you want to use. For instance, you may want to use (and may have to use) a primary care doctor from the HMO but decide to go out of network for a cardiologist at a higher cost to you than a cardiologist in the HMO. You can make this decision for each episode of care.

You may even have a triple choice plan, where you can get care in the HMO (no extra cost), get care in the PPO network (some out-of-pocket costs), or go outside of both the HMO and PPO to another health care provider (yet higher out-of-pocket costs).

Even though a POS lets you go to a non-network doctor, it does not erase the basic rules of managed care. The primary care physician can still be a player here. Make sure to check whether there are any limitations on services not authorized by a primary care physician.

Specialty HMOs and "Carve-Outs"

Sometimes mental health and substance abuse treatment, dental and vision care, and pharmacy benefits are separated from the basic health plan. Some plans allow you to choose whether you want that coverage and are willing to pay a separate premium for it, as is often the case in dental or vision. Some offer this coverage under the umbrella of the rest of the plan, as is often the case with mental health and substance abuse care, but those services are provided by separate plans. Such plans often have special requirements, especially for referrals.

Healthspeak
Carve-outs are medical services that are separated from the rest of the arrangements and contracted for separately. Medical-surgical services may also be carved out from the basic plan. *Specialty HMOs* are set up exactly like HMOs except they specialize in a particular set of health issues, like dental or mental health. They must meet state requirements for HMOs.

There may be extra steps to using these benefits, different from the way you usually use your plan. Check to see which benefits may be carve-outs and make sure you know the drill for getting care:

➤ Sometimes mental health plans require a referral from the primary care doctor to the psychiatrist or appropriate counselor.

➤ Telephone numbers for getting services or information may be different from the rest of your plan.

➤ Often the charges to you are different from those in the rest of the plan.

➤ The list of participating physicians may also be different. There are also separate lists for counselors, social workers, and dentists.

Who Is Looking Over My (and My Doctor's) Shoulder?

Someone in the health plan is always watching how you use the plan and how your doctor treats his patients. The plan also has the power to limit or deny payment for treatment. One way this is done is through *utilization review (UR)* or *utilization management (UM)*. UR/UM, or the process of reviewing treatments to assess their appropriateness, is key to keeping cost under control for managed care organizations. UR/UM is also used to preauthorize the next step in medical care, whether that is a set of lab tests, hospitalization, or an operation. This deliberate hurdle is a key part of the business practices of managed care plans, and it is a major part of developing a game plan for serious, costly illness.

In a nutshell, UR is used to make the decision that the care the patient is about to receive is necessary and appropriate—the two big guns for deciding whether your care will be okayed by the plan. UM is a process to review care after it is received. Now your experience and that of other patients is combined to develop a picture of how doctors and other health care providers deliver care—their practice patterns—and come up with appropriate guidelines.

Healthspeak

Utilization review or *utilization management* is a practice in which teams of doctors, nurses, and other health care professionals review the treatment history of patients in order to evaluate the appropriateness of their health care treatment. UR is usually before treatment begins, and UM is review after it has been received.

Each organization has different rules to this game. Some managed care plans have very strict guidelines. If you want to see a specialist and your doctor thinks you should see a specialist, the doctor may have to call the UR department before making the referral. Sometimes it's looser. The doctor refers you to a specialist by filling out the referral form you take to the specialist, but still must call UR for more extraordinary procedures.

However UR/UM is organized, it is the part of managed care that your doctor and often his office staff battles on your behalf. But it can also take time. Ask your doctor and his staff how long it can take. Sometimes it can take 7 to 10 days to hear back on nonemergencies.

Now you see why you and your doctor are not alone in the examining room. Somewhere just out of sight there are hundreds of people thinking about what you and your doctor want and whether or not it's good for you—and them.

The Least You Need to Know

➤ Know whether you have an HMO, PPO, or POS plan. Knowing what you have will guide what you do and what you expect from your plan.

➤ Managed care has become more common because it promised and delivered a stopper in yearly health premium increases.

➤ Every managed care plan has rules for using its services, particularly referrals. These rules are the cornerstone of how these plans control cost.

➤ Some services such as mental health and substance abuse, dental, vision, and pharmacy are carve-outs and sometimes have their own rules, copayment (see Chapter 5), and telephone numbers. Make sure you know the rules and numbers if they are different from the rest of your plan.

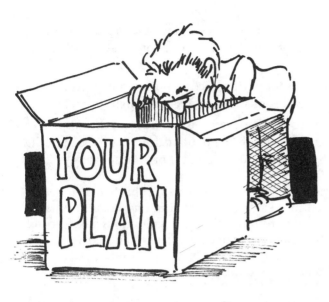

Chapter 2

Your Plan from the Inside Out

In This Chapter

➤ It's just business

➤ "B" team or all-stars: your health care providers

➤ Who signs the checks

➤ You and your doctor, but maybe not forever

➤ Big changes for hospitals, too

The most overworked metaphor in business is the sports team. Real estate has its all-star sales teams, stockbrokers have the Big Game, and some company is always trying to get a level playing field. In spite of that, we'll continue to exploit the sports metaphor to explain managed care because it has been so wholeheartedly embraced by the health care industry.

Before managed care, medicine was like sandlot ball: a few players, a few basic rules, and the guy with the bat (the patient) got to choose the team. Now, your health care rests in a managed care plan that seems to resemble a professional sports team:

➤ You are a member of the team, but your team is the plan—doctors, hospitals, managers, reviewers, marketers, stockholders—not just you and your doctor.

➤ Your contract is with your managed care team. If your doctor leaves, it's only one member of the team leaving. You stay with the team. You don't leave with your buddy.

➤ There are as many different formulas for paying doctors as there are sports contracts. Sometimes they may affect your care. Sometimes you have the right to find out.

➤ They moved the stadium. The focus of health care has moved from the hospital to the health plan. This is happening across the board, no matter what type of health plan you have. The emphasis is on outpatient care and shorter hospital stays.

Competition is the name of the game played by investor-owned, publicly traded health care corporations and large, not-for-profit medical service institutions. Private capital markets are the funders for public and nonprofit health care organizations alike. Doctors now answer to large organizations with their own game plans and financial risks.

May the Market Force Be with You

Managed care plans sell a product line: their supply of networks of doctors and hospitals, its affiliations or contracts with rehab and specialty centers, and its ability and expertise in managing care and costs. Its income is based on its ability to sell enough of this to stay in business or turn a profit and provide value for shareholders for the for-profit plans.

Healthspeak
Managed care plans can be *not-for-profit* or *for-profit*. Nonprofit plans don't have shareholders; for-profits do. Managed care plans can be owned by charities, insurance companies, employers, hospitals, or groups of physicians.

Why is it important to know about the business side of managed care?

➤ You need to know how to wade through the jargon and advertising to understand what your plan really delivers.

➤ You need to be able to judge if your plan can provide the type of care you need.

➤ You want to know what incentives the plan has to provide good care. This will help you become your own best advocate in a world of competing pressures.

Managed care affects the practice of medicine everywhere, from the small labs in your pediatrician's building to the large academic hospitals 20 miles away. Because you are now a member of the team rather than a lone player, you need to know why the team works the way it does. One way to find out is to look at how plans pick doctors and how they pay them.

Eenie, Meenie, Minie, Moe: How They Pick Doctors

For both HMOs and PPOs, choosing doctors—how many and what kind—is the plan's core business decision. Whatever calculations they use, their mix of doctors, hospitals, and specialized services is where their bread is buttered.

Let's use a couple of hypothetical health plans—the ACHES Plan and the PANES Plan (they'll appear throughout the book) to show how this works. For instance, the ACHES Plan may decide that four immunologists is the right number, while the PANES Plan decides that two is enough. If PANES expands its service area, they may increase the number to five. Or they may decide to contract with a network of primary care doctors whose practice is owned by a local hospital, and then funnel patients to the hospital at a discounted fee. There are many variations to putting together the services of a managed care plan, enough to spawn an entire industry that reconfigures physician practices and negotiates contracts among everyone involved in the plan.

House Call

Your managed care plan is neither your best friend nor a religion: It's a business. Keep this in mind to adjust your expectations for both service and quality. Some knowledge of the business side may be useful if you think your care is being compromised and you want to complain to the state or start legal proceedings.

Doctors' willingness to affiliate with managed care plans has increased dramatically since 1991. New managed care plans or plans new to an area often sign up any doctor willing to accept their payment arrangement so they can make inroads into a market.

Doctors can be employees of an HMO or employees of the staffing group that services the HMO. They have salaries and occasionally bonuses. They are subject to usual recruitment, hiring, and firing of any company. Doctors can also contract with a network, or with an HMO, to provide services for a certain amount of money per patient (capitation) or per visit (fee-for-service). In that case, they are not employees of the network.

Preferred provider organizations (PPOs) give discounts for volume purchases—discounts the consumer loses when they buy services from non-PPO providers. These networks, or the networks they contract with, discount their prices for medical services in exchange for the insurer routing their enrollees to them. As a result, the enrollees pay less than they would a non-network provider.

In some ways, it's like buying a set of dishes. Often the physician networks provide a complete service of primary care doctors and specialists. But sometimes certain specialists and more often subspecialists have to be special ordered.

Now comes the tricky part: picking high-quality doctors. Or is it? If you read or listen to the ads, every managed care plan has the top ten doctors in town. Let's take a closer look at some of those claims, because each plan has a different way of deciding what is quality.

There is no absolute standard. The National Commission on Quality Assurance (NCQA), a private organization that examines HMOs, looks to see if HMOs check out the physician's credentials (for more on doctor credentials, see Chapter 6).

NCQA also asks if the plan investigates the training and experience of the doctors that it signs, looks for a history of malpractice or fraud, and tracks the performance of its doctors. This standard is a little different than the usual credentialing by hospitals, which check if hospital privileges were revoked, if there are disciplinary actions against the doctor, or if the doctors' licenses were revoked. Sometimes PPOs use credentialing similar to that of hospitals.

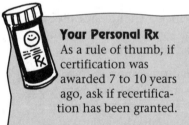

Healthspeak
Board-certified doctors or other health care professionals have passed a test given by their national specialty organization. *Board-eligible* doctors may be awaiting their exam results or may have completed approved training and are waiting to take the exams.

Your Personal Rx
As a rule of thumb, if certification was awarded 7 to 10 years ago, ask if recertification has been granted.

Probably the biggest claim made by managed care plans in their pitch to employers and individuals is that their physicians are *board-certified* or *board-eligible*.

Board certification is the floor in most managed care plans—and a useful one at that. It weeds out those who could not pass the tests. This should also be the floor for looking at quality in a plan. Anyone with a license can practice in any specialty, but a board-certified doctor is one who has completed the appropriate training for the specialty and passed the test.

Some specialties require recertification, which means that their specialists must take another test every few years. However, don't expect this of every board-certified doctor. Some who were practicing before the specialty organization decided to test for recertification may not in fact have to be retested. They are considered to be "grandfathered," exempt from needing retesting by virtue of their experience. The amount of time in practice in order to be grandfathered varies depending on the specialty.

Your Health Care Team

The more you know about the health care professionals available to you, the better you will be able to advocate for your best care. Your plan will probably include a number of health care professionals in addition to your doctor, nurse, and dentist.

You may have the option of choosing a number of *mid-level health care professionals* for primary and other care. Mid-level health care professionals may be called nurse practitioners, nurse-midwives, physician assistants, and certified registered nurse-anesthetists.

While these professionals must practice with or under the supervision of a physician, they make many patient management decisions on their own.

You will also generally have a choice between a standard M.D. or an *osteopathic physician* (with a D.O., not an M.D., after his or her name). An osteopathic physician's training places special emphasis on the relationship between the musculoskeletal system and the body's other systems.

Most health care plans also cover treatment by a *chiropractor* for certain conditions or injuries. A chiropractor treats disorders based on the theory that they are caused by interference with nerve function, and uses manipulation of the body joints and the spine to restore normal function.

Your plan may deliver mental health services using a variety of professionals. Psychiatrists are M.D.s and can order prescription drugs. Some psychologists, who are not M.D.s, receive additional training so they can prescribe drugs as well. Mental health services may also be delivered by social workers and psychiatric nurses, as well as primary care physicians.

Your plan is also likely to enroll registered dieticians, who are specialists in the use of proper, balanced diet to promote health. Dieticians can be helpful in the management of many chronic conditions. Your plan may also enroll audiology (hearing) services and speech therapy providers.

The Almighty Dollar: How Your Doctors Are Paid

Let's tackle the dreaded "C" word: capitation. This is the type of payment that is often mentioned in managed care horror stories about doctors not seeing patients or detrimentally limiting care.

Doctors can be paid a fee each time a service is performed or on a capitated basis. Capitated payments are usually a certain amount per month per health plan member enrolled with that doctor. A primary care physician in a capitated plan may be paid $30 per month per member signed up with her, whether you see her five times in a month or not at all. She is paid by the head, not by the visit or procedure.

If your doctor receives capitated payments from the managed care plan, he gets a fixed amount of money per month for each patient signed up with him. There is a financial incentive to undertreat patients who need more services.

Your Personal Rx
Why do you need to know something about how doctors are paid? It is one of the major changes in how health care is paid for, and it may affect how often and how much time your doctor spends with you. Some states and the American Association of Health Plans (AAHP), a managed care trade group, require the plan to answer members' questions about physician reimbursement.

17

And other questions pop up. For instance, if Doctor Fibula receives $20 per person per month from the ACHES Plan, and $50 from PANES plan, will he spend less time and effort on the ACHES members?

But there is also a financial incentive to prevent illness and keep you healthy. Keeping you healthy may mean emphasizing preventive services to head off lots of trips to the doctor or specialist. Other incentives to your doctor to keep you healthy include professional ethics and the possibility of malpractice suits.

Capitation is the payment of choice for primary care doctors and specialists in large markets where there is intense competition among plans. Beyond establishing a certain payment per head, payment arrangements can get very creative. Capitation may not be used alone; bonuses and other monetary incentives are often used.

Managed care plans sometimes take into account their measures of quality when they choose bonus and incentive arrangements. These measurements include the following:

➤ Member satisfaction

➤ Rate that patients transfer to other doctors

➤ Results of medical charts reviews

➤ Compliance with the other plan standards

Plans may also consider things like office procedures, hours, patient management, and the use of specialists and emergency rooms.

Sound a bit complicated? Let's add another dimension. Many HMOs have different payment arrangements with different doctors in their plans. Under one type of arrangement, the plan withholds a certain percentage of a doctor's fees until the end of an accounting period. If her total medical expenses are lower than the organization's target amount, she gets her withheld fees.

Does capitation have an effect on how medicine is practiced? Yes. But how much of an effect really varies. Doctors who take a number of managed care plans may be less affected by one plan's payment arrangement than a doctor who takes only a few. Some doctors refuse to participate in capitated plans. The bottom line is that good compensation arrangements are important to offset the limiting of services under a pure capitation arrangement.

It's Hard to Say Goodbye: When Your Doctor Leaves Your Plan

You may have signed up with a managed care plan because you wanted to go to Dr. Bee. That doesn't mean he'll be there after you join.

House Call

Managed care plans rate doctor selection and retention as very important to their success. Keep this in mind when you look at new plans. The National Commission on Quality Assurance (NCQA) also looks at what percentage of doctors leave the plan each year when it certifies HMOs.

Physicians can be fired or quit from staff model HMOs just like any other employee. Or they can resign or be dropped from IPAs and PPOs. If you want to continue with your doctor, you will have to change plans. There is no guarantee that your doctor will stay with the plan as long as you do.

Remember, one of the major concepts of managed care is that you are a member of the plan. You get your health care through the plan, of which your doctor is one of a cast of hundreds. Even though you may intend to change plans and follow him, you may not be able to do that for a number of months.

Doctors move on and off provider networks and PPO lists in sometimes unpredictable ways. Changes in reimbursement schedules can sometimes lead to wholesale abandonment of plans by doctors, and reevaluation of practice patterns can lead to doctors being removed from plans.

You are not sent an announcement that your doctor has left the plan. Sometimes the first you know your doctor has left your plan is when you see a note at the receptionist's desk. Some contracts forbid doctors to contact patients to inform them they have been dropped from the plan.

Your Personal Rx

When you are choosing a plan, make sure you have a couple of doctors you would use in case your doctor leaves. Ask your previous doctor for a recommendation to another doctor, but also check with other plan members—friends, relatives, or coworkers—for their suggestions.

This can be terribly frustrating to the patient. If you have not seen a particular doctor lately, check to see if she is still with your plan before your schedule an appointment.

Hospitals and Managed Care

Hospitals look and act differently than before managed care became such a force. Hospitals —their personnel and facilities—are costly to maintain. By emphasizing outpatient care and free-standing facilities, like labs and urgent care centers, managed care has a powerful influence on hospitals. They are no longer the center of the health care system but on the periphery. Managed care has changed who owns them, what they do, and how they are paid.

You may be able to better understand what is happening to hospitals by visualizing a tree. First you have the trunk, your basic local hospital that's been around for 50 years. In order to survive the intense competition for patients and referrals, it branches into other areas like home health care and pharmacies. It affiliates with other hospitals. It sheds costly expenditures like support and business services and buys them on a contract basis.

The move to managed care has also put pressure on hospitals to be part of *integrated delivery systems*. Hospitals are also merging with other hospitals, for-profit hospitals are buying not-for-profit hospitals, and many are buying primary care practices.

Healthspeak

An *integrated delivery system* combines health care providers like hospitals, doctors and other medical staff, and professionals under one organizational structure to provide a broad spectrum of health care services. They are often contracted as one entity to several different health plans.

Your Personal Rx

If you are changing plans (or your employer is changing for you) and you have a special condition that is treated at a teaching hospital, check whether the hospital is in your plan. Check your plan's other hospitals and their affiliations with other teaching hospitals. Remember, there is no guarantee your plan will continue with that hospital or that your employer will continue with that plan.

Hospitals can be paid on a capitation basis just like doctors. They can get paid a lump sum per day the member is in the hospital. If you are kept there longer, it costs the hospital more. If they cut back, they get to keep the rest. There are just as many ways to configure hospital capitation as doctor capitation. It represents a lot of money to both the hospital and the doctors in the system.

What all this activity means to the consumer is that the choice of hospital is very limited. Hospitalization means big bucks, and keeping a lid on the costs has produced a very complicated, restrictive environment. The hospital (or hospital system) that gives your doctors admitting privileges, that meets cost targets, and that meets certain quality goals of the managed care plan is where you go.

What has happened to the crème de la crème, the teaching hospital? This is often the care center for the most severely ill or those with rare diseases. Right now they are going through mergers, acquisitions, and are being sold to for-profit hospital chains.

Costs are higher at teaching hospitals, in part because they treat high-cost patients. Managed care plans are but one pressure, albeit a major pressure, on teaching hospitals to put the lid on cost. The federal government and states are also putting the brakes on for spending for health.

The effect on you, the consumer, is that being treated at a teaching hospital may be a very difficult proposition. You may be frozen out of care at a teaching hospital by your health plan's contract with other hospitals. (See Chapters 17 and 18 for more information on very specialized care).

However, many managed care plans are affiliated with teaching hospitals. Your plan may make available to you a number of hospitals with university medical school affiliations not unlike the hospital you have in mind. Keep in mind that this is a very volatile situation, and one that bears watching.

The Least You Need to Know

➤ You are now a member of the managed care team, a host of people responsible for the delivery and financing of your health care. The doctor-patient duet no longer exists.

➤ There are many ways managed care plans pay doctors, hospitals, and others who provide care for you. Sometimes they can affect your care; other times they won't.

➤ Board certification is required of doctors hired by most managed care plans. Board certification alone won't differentiate one plan's quality from another, but it is a floor, and a good one at that.

➤ The mix of hospitals, doctors, and other health care providers is the core of the managed care business. Make sure the mix provides the services you need.

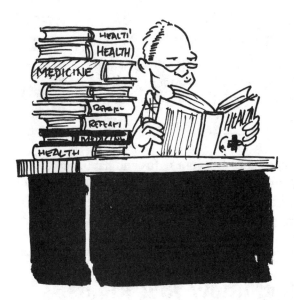

Chapter 3

The Informed Consumer Gets the Best Health Care

In This Chapter

➤ Knowing your health care rights

➤ Organizing your records

➤ Keeping track of special medical events

Do you keep lists everywhere on how to manage your time, your life, and your job? Are your drawers stuffed with booklets on how to improve your health, finances, and looks? Is your computer aching under the strain of new software that promises to simplify your life? You may be suffering from Informed Consumer Syndrome. It seems that everybody expects you to be an informed consumer, from the IRS to the county recycling center to your bank. One difference: Being an informed health care consumer is not only essential; it could quite literally be a lifesaver.

In the past, your employer, the government, and the health care system treated you only as a patient. Now they all expect and rely on you to be a consumer. What's the difference? A patient is passive, and a consumer is active. A patient is given care, a consumer buys care. You are responsible for health care choices. You are expected to respond to mountains of information on healthy living, know how to choose and use your health care plan, and deal with any health problems you may (or may in the future) have. Every interaction with the health care system requires you to make decisions.

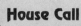

House Call

Remember: You are the one paying for your health care coverage, whether it comes directly from your bank account or from the wages your employer would otherwise have paid you. Understand your rights and your coverage to get the most for *your* money.

Being an informed health care consumer means knowing your rights and having access to your medical records. It means getting your hands on the essential information when you need it. And it means knowing how to use the power of information on your behalf.

We could spend days setting up lists of things you must know, should know, and are in great peril if you don't know. But we know from experience that the only way to keep things from ending up in the junk drawer is to keep them simple.

There Is Power in Knowledge: Know Your Rights

The first thing you have to know is that when you are enrolled in a health care coverage plan, you acquire certain rights. This is true whether the coverage comes with your paycheck or you pay for it on your own. Though the letters and brochures you receive from your employer or health plan may look boring and tedious, hold on to them. You never know when you (or your lawyer) may need to use them.

Your Right to Information

Employer-sponsored health care plans must meet certain rules set out by the federal government in the Internal Revenue Code (IRC) and the Employee Retirement Income Security Act (ERISA). ERISA provides you with important protections for any type of benefit your employer may offer, including pensions, various types of insurance, vacation pay, sick pay, and severance pay. Medicare (Chapter 8) and Medicaid (Chapter 10) offer still other protections.

Assume any benefit your employer offers to its employees has to obey ERISA rules. Federal, state, and local government employees have different rights and protections—in some cases—from those available to private-sector employees. These vary by level of government and by state. See your human resources office if you have questions about the rights that apply to you.

Your health plan must be in writing and communicated appropriately to plan *participants* and their *beneficiaries*. That means you have to be informed in writing that the plan exists and what it does for you. The *plan administrator* who does not do so risks criminal and civil sanctions.

You have a right to certain types of information from the plan, some general and some specific to your situation:

➤ The health plan must furnish you a description, called a Summary Plan Description (SPD), written in a way that the average plan participant or beneficiary can understand. That means you! Among other things, the SPD has to describe the benefits the plan provides and how you get them.

➤ The information in the SPD may not give you everything you need. In that case, you can look at your plan's contract for health care coverage and services. This is usually a very large document and is not handed out to everyone. You can find the contract in the plan administrator's office. Check with your human resources or personnel departments.

➤ If you file a claim for benefits and it is denied, you have a right to be informed of the reasons. The explanation (called an Explanation of Benefits or EOB), shown on the following page, must be in writing and written in a way you can understand. It can't be all "legalese." The plan is also required to give you a reasonable chance to appeal a benefit denial, and you may have the right to sue the plan, the employer, or both in court (more on this in Chapters 23 and 24).

➤ You may also have the right to certain types of plan information and benefits when your own individual circumstances change (you get married, have a baby, divorce, and so on). We discuss these further in Chapter 7.

Healthspeak
A plan *participant* or *beneficiary* is an employee or dependent of that employee who is receiving benefits or who is eligible to receive benefits from an employee benefit plan. The *plan administrator* is the person or firm designated by your health plan or employer to handle day-to-day details of record keeping, claims handling, and filing of reports.

Your Personal Rx
If you don't understand the Summary Plan Description (SPD), you have a right to ask questions. The SPD also has to be updated if the plan is changed.

When you have questions about your benefits or need to resolve a dispute, go to your employer, not the insurance company that underwrites or administers the plan. Your employer usually has the legal obligation to answer your questions. The company, on the other hand, can have many plans tailored to the needs of different employers and often isn't of much use when you have a question.

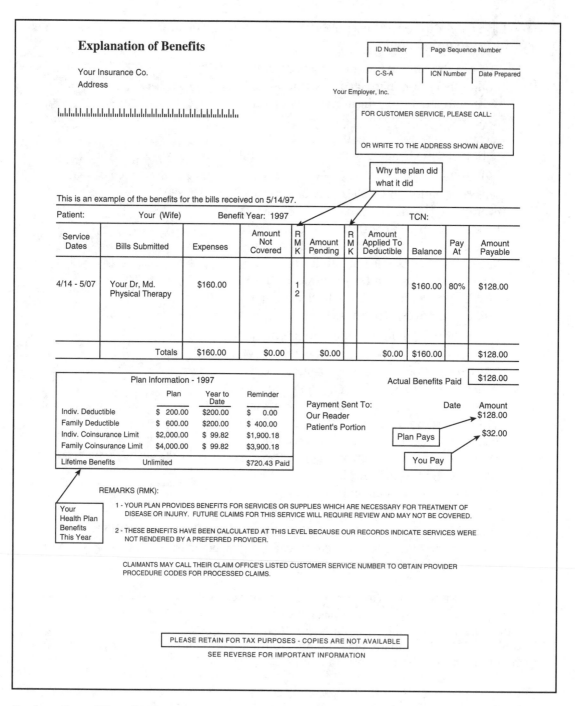

Explanation of Benefits form.

House Call

Don't assume a plan is insured—and therefore subject to state laws governing insurance plans—just because you send claim forms to an insurance company. Many insurance companies operate self-insured plans for employers under administrative-services-only contracts. In a self-insured plan, the employer pays for the claims out of its revenues as they occur. The insurance company handles only the plan's paperwork; it doesn't insure the plan.

Your Right to Coverage

Employers don't have to offer health care plans. If they do, they don't have to offer coverage for dependents. They are also not required to cover everybody they employ. But, if they do offer coverage they have certain responsibilities.

Until now, insurers were able to exclude certain people in a group based on their health history, or even refuse to cover whole groups because the employer's industry or the health of one or more potential participants was considered too risky. But under a new federal law, effective for most plans in 1998 (more on this in Chapter 7), insurance carriers can't refuse group coverage to employers—or refuse to cover individual employees in a group—based on their...

➤ Health

➤ Past use of health care

➤ Evidence of insurability

➤ Disability

➤ Medical conditions

➤ Medical history

➤ Genetic information

Group plans also cannot set different enrollment or coverage requirements, nor can they charge you more for your coverage based on these criteria. Insurers also have to renew the policies of any employers who ask them without regard to these criteria. However, plans and insurers are free to continue to charge fees and premiums based on the past cost of covering a given group. So, even if coverage is available, there is no guarantee it will continue to be affordable.

Healthspeak
Genetic information concerns genes, gene products, and inherited characteristics of an individual or a family member. Genetic information can suggest your chances of getting a disease or passing it on to your child.

Your Right to Use Your Benefits

Sometimes people are afraid of being fired or otherwise discriminated against if they (or a member of their family) get sick. They may forgo getting treatment for a physical or mental condition. Or they may pay for treatment out of their own pockets because they fear their employer can fire or make trouble for them if they file claims.

Federal law protects you against such reprisals. You or your family cannot be hurt in any way for exercising your rights to benefits the plan already provides to you. That means the employer can't fire you either because you have filed claims, or because the employer is afraid you will do so.

House Call

If you become ill or disabled, your job is protected under the Americans with Disabilities Act. You can lose your job only if you can't perform its essential functions, with or without reasonable accommodations to your situation. But addiction to illegal drugs is not a protected disability, so you could lose your job even if you are in treatment.

Get Your Medical Records

Do any of these situations ring a bell?

You have changed jobs, and with your new paycheck comes a new health plan and the need to choose a new doctor. Your employer has offered you a relocation package you can't resist—but you can't take your old doctor with you! You have a chronic health condition and you wonder if you would benefit from recent medical advances in managing it, or perhaps you want to be prepared in case of an emergency. You are applying for health or life insurance and are asked to authorize release of your medical history (more on releases in Chapter 22). You are being billed for something you were positive your insurance should have covered. Your child wants to go to that fabulous tennis camp the city runs in the summer.

What do these situations have in common?

You need your medical records. What these records include is discussed in detail in Chapter 22, but here we want you to recognize that these records are an important part of your household files. And we don't just mean the receipts and EOBs (treat those like you would your canceled checks or tax returns). We mean the actual medical stuff that deals with the condition of your body parts.

Getting your medical records is a not a simple, one-time event. Unless you have spent your entire life in one staff model HMO, a nice, neat file does not move from office to office each time you encounter the health system. Each physician you have seen or health plan you have belonged to most likely has only records on treatment received there and is obligated to send only those records to whomever you tell it to.

You need to get health files for all members of the family, including information on immunizations, major illnesses, and hospitals where you or your family were treated. If you have the dates and places of hospitalizations, you can lead your doctor to records you may have misplaced or never had. People often forget what hospital they were at many years ago, and the hospital names are always changing. If you need records from a long-ago hospital stay, call or write the medical records department of that facility, giving as much information as you can. If you are missing any of your children's immunization records, make a copy at their school from their school records if you can't get them from your doctor.

If you go to a physician other than your primary care doctor, ask for records after the visit. Most specialists will write a letter to your primary care doctor explaining their opinion of your case; this letter will usually make more sense to you than notes written in medical lingo and abbreviations. But paperwork can fall through the cracks. If your primary care doctor does not get that letter in a reasonable period of time, ask the specialist for it or at least for a copy of her notes to give your primary care doctor. Ask for records after each hospital visit. If you rarely get medical care and find it hard to remember to get records, connect it to a milestone, like a birthday or anniversary, and make a point to get them at that time each year.

When asking for your medical records, remember that the information is legally yours, but the actual files belong to the hospital, doctor, or insurer. Some states give you the right to see your medical records if you ask, but others don't (more in Chapter 22). You may receive an actual copy, or you may get a summary. You will usually have to pay for copying, but the charges are usually modest.

Coping with Information Overload

One of the tricks of keeping medical records is not to lose them or mix them up with report cards and bank statements. Try a three-ring binder you can keep in a drawer, or a simple folder with pockets (some bright color you can find when you need it). Keep a notebook with information about your health plan. Plans change from year to year. You are supposed to receive a booklet or a set of papers (addendum) in the mail on changes to your plan. Review it carefully and keep it with your health plan papers. If you keep a three-ring binder, put it in the front part of your plan so you keep those changes in mind when you have to use your plan.

Your Personal Rx
Check with your employee benefits manager or your insurance agent from time to time to make sure that you haven't missed any materials, especially if you anticipate a major procedure or an addition to your family. And if you have a complaint, don't wait—state it right away.

Authorization for Release of Medical Information

I authorize

_____
Name of sending person, agency or institution

_____
Address

_____
City   State   Zip

to release to

_____
Name of receiving person, agency or institution

_____
Address

_____
City   State   Zip

the following information: (Information to be released must be clearly specified)

_____

in regard to _____   _____
              Name of patient at time of treatment   Medical Record No.

_____   (_____) _____   for the purpose of _____
Date of birth   Pt's day phone number

_____

I understand that I may revoke this consent at any time except to the extent that action has been taken based on this authorization. I also understand that this authorization shall expire, without my express revocation, three months from the date written below.

_____   _____
Signature of patient or responsible person   Date

_____
Witness

If this release pertains to alcohol or drug abuse information, please note that:

This information has been disclosed to you from records whose confidentiality is protected by Federal law. Federal regulation (42 C.F.R. Part 2) prohibits you from making further disclosure of it without the specific written consent of the patient to whom it pertains, or as otherwise permitted by such regulations. A general authorization for the release of medical or other information is NOT sufficient for this purpose.

Release of Records form.

Hang On to Your Handbook

You always receive a members' handbook, which gives a "quick read" of your rights, benefits, and vital telephone numbers. Make sure you keep this item handy. It's usually small enough to carry in a purse or briefcase, so it's easy to take to the doctor or hospital with you. Sometimes that's the downside: It's easy to slide under the front seat of the car or on top of the phone books. But wherever you put it, keep in mind that it's one of your most important reference books and can save you a lot of time (and sometimes heartache) if you know where it is.

The member handbook also gives you information on crucial parts of the plan, such as what you need to do for referrals or what to do in emergencies. Make some notes, and maybe use some sticky note pads for sections you'll use often. And if you make a run to the emergency room, be sure to take your members' guide with you.

House Call

Why do you need to take the member handbook to visit a doctor in your plan? Some doctors belong to only a few plans and may know what your plan allows. Others belong to many plans and don't have a clue, aren't up to date, or can make critical mistakes. It's a good way to double-check services and save money, too.

Getting Answers from Member Services

Now, let's talk about information you request from the plan. One of the "rules" of joining any health plan is to ask lots of questions when you join so that you don't get caught in a bind later. The first place to start is with member services, who are trained to respond (or forward) most questions about the health plan.

Remember: There are no stupid questions, just mushy answers. Sometimes you have to be assertive and persistent. Your objective is to get questions answered to *your* satisfaction, not theirs. If the person you talk to is unable to answer adequately, ask to speak to a supervisor. If you have trouble understanding the information given to you, ask them to repeat it or send written confirmation or other plan information that would shed light on your question.

Your Personal Rx

It pays to keep track of information given to you by member services in response to your questions—even if they are short notes to yourself. Try to date them and get the name of the person giving you information. This can help you later if you relied on the information and it was wrong.

Member services is also the first place that must be contacted if you want to complain about your care, follow up on a claim that was denied by the plan, or file a grievance. They are sometimes required by law or by the terms of the plan to answer within a certain amount of time (more in Chapter 23).

Caution

If you do record your call, tell the person to whom you are talking that you are doing so, or you could be violating the law. Make sure you turn on the recorder before the call to get the whole call and record the other person's permission.

If you are unhappy with your managed care plan's response to your questions or its response to requests for services, keep a log of those phone calls. If you decide to lodge a complaint or take your complaint up the supervisory line, a record adds to your credibility and gives you some evidence of poor or questionable services.

You may want to record your calls with your plan. This is most useful if the subject matter is complicated or if you are at odds with your plan. Sometimes it is difficult to remember all the information. Your notes can be sketchy, especially if, as is often the case, colleagues are walking in and out of your office or the kids are yelling in the background.

But remember that recording calls without the other person's permission is generally illegal.

Special Events and Chronic Illnesses

Now that you are considered a "partner" in your own care, be prepared to take an active role in making decisions about the course of your treatment. One of the ways to do this is to keep a list of questions that you can update as they occur to you. Keep it where you spend a lot of time so that you don't put off writing them down. Preferably, for the sake of confidentiality, keep it at home.

Special events like pregnancy or severe or chronic illnesses require a vigilant approach to keeping track of your medical files. Keep a record of dates of treatments and medications. If you have an ongoing problem, record dates and times episodes occur. Most doctors we talked to said that patients do a good job of recording dates and times of episodes but have a more difficult time describing and writing down symptoms.

Many doctors and patients told us that support groups and national organizations are absolutely key in understanding a chronic condition and keeping up with the latest treatments. They are often your window on the latest developments and can be an advocate in winding your way through the process of getting good care.

House Call

Some health plans and hospitals sponsor support groups. Your specialist often knows what is available locally. Health plan newsletters also list support group meetings.

The storytelling that goes on in support groups is a powerful tool. Not only does it provide comfort and sharing at a time when you often feel alone, it also provides a wealth of information on what to expect during the course of an illness and how to deal with health plans and health care providers.

The Least You Need to Know

➤ Be aware of your rights as a member of a health plan. Hold on to those special brochures like the Summary Plan Description (SPD) and changes to the plans (amendments). In the best of worlds, you need them only for reference. In the worst of worlds, you need them to assert your rights.

➤ Make your medical records *your* records. Don't rely on them being sent from one health care plan, or one physician, to the next. Get copies, and keep them where you can find them.

➤ Try to keep tabs on information that you asked for from the plan. A note with the date, the person you talked to, and (briefly) what was said is fine.

➤ Special events like pregnancy and surgeries require more vigilance. Keep records of dates, treatments, and medications.

➤ If you have a chronic condition, join national support groups for the latest on treatments, what to expect, and what you need to know.

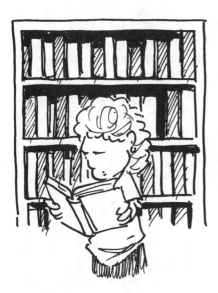

The Home Health Bookshelf

Everyone should have a couple of health care books at home. If you take out a splinter or need to answer a question about your sleepless baby, it's useful and comforting to keep a few essential health books and resources.

But managed care has created new expectations that go beyond splinter removal proficiency. You are expected to be health literate. This means the onus is on you to be responsible for interpreting and understanding all sorts of instructions, from how to use your health plan to the cautions on your prescription. There is a shift of perspective from patient to consumer—the type of consumer who reads and understands the warranties.

If you fall skateboarding down your driveway, you are expected to know why your shoulder injury is not an emergency, and whether the pain medication your doctor prescribed interacts with your cholesterol medication. And if you plan to try it again, you may want to find out if your health plan pays for extra splints.

Why is it important to have a grasp of how to hunt down and use medical information?

➤ Your plan counts on your ability to make informed choices, whether about your doctors, your treatments, or even about which benefits you need. Your doctor is making many choices, too, and cost containment plays a part. You have to have the information to ask the questions that can enhance or save your life.

➤ You need the power of information if you want to say "no" to your doctor's or health plan's recommendations, or force them to say "yes" to your ideas. When facing a bureaucracy, you must be prepared to be your own advocate.

House Call

One family had a newborn who required extensive heart and kidney testing. The father forced the managed care plan's hand by knowing neonatal units in their area far more capable of the specialized testing he needed than those under the plan. He started with his public library, worked his way to local medical schools, and scanned the Internet. He was firm in his commitment (and aggressive with the plan) to get tests at the most qualified center. You may not be armed and dangerous, but you can be armed and intelligent.

➤ You may have to work fast. We all know of cases where an elderly parent takes a turn for the worse and develops multiple health problems. Or an injury leads to complications, and you have to figure out a new track to recovery. Decisions must be made within a short amount of time, and you want to be fully informed to make the best ones possible.

A home health bookshelf is the first step to becoming an informed consumer. Knowing how to find the other information you need is the next step.

At Your Fingertips

Perhaps your health care bookshelf consists of only a dog-eared copy of an old first-aid book. Or perhaps you are the neighborhood's medical librarian-in-residence, with the largest lending library this side of the local med school. Whichever one describes you, follow these three rules to stock your health care bookshelf:

➤ Make sure the books give basic information that helps anyone who must react to health care situations in your house: yourself, older children, baby-sitters, caretakers, or relatives.

➤ Find books that are easy to read. You can get medical school textbooks, if that's your preference, but these are generally not the best basic references for everyday use.

Books with pictures are good, and make sure the book or books you choose have good indexes.

➤ Put the books in a convenient place—maybe with the phone books, cookbooks, or any set of reading materials that are used often. No one should need to hunt them down.

Some HMOs give out, or offer at a reduced rate, books about common health problems. Some offer instructions on what to do if you suffer from certain symptoms and when to call the doctor or go to the emergency room. These are good to have around, and are usually written and illustrated in such a way that older children or baby-sitters can read and understand them.

They also serve another very important purpose: They provide a vocabulary to use when you talk to your managed care organization's advice line or urgent care line (see Chapter 14 for more on urgent care). There are key words and phrases that they use to make decisions, and they are probably the same or similar to those used in the book or books they provide.

If you want more particulars than you find in your basic health care books, there is a whole industry at your beck and call. You can feed your curiosity or even take up a new hobby by exploring the wealth of health information in CD-ROMs, magazines, and newsletters. Plan newsletters also provide lists of events and helpful advice endorsed by the plan.

Everyone is writing about health. We've seen articles on stress and repetitive motion injuries, high blood pressure, health insurance, and emergency services in every kind of magazine. Sometimes half the articles in women's magazines are devoted to health.

The problem with giving them a lot of weight is that it's difficult to judge the reliability of the information. But they can provide a good starting point for asking questions about your plan's coverage and services.

> **Your Personal Rx**
> If you have what we call "milestones," events such as pregnancy, surgery, or a new diagnosis for a chronic condition, get a basic but comprehensive book on the topic for your health care bookshelf. Holding on to pamphlets from your doctor's office sometimes provides enough material, but they often get scattered or tossed out.

Our friend Jane read an article touting a new, FDA-approved test for cervical cancer in a recent local business magazine. She recalled reading an article in a popular women's magazine about the 20 to 30 percent false negatives on pap smears that occur each year, which can lead women to falsely believe they are cancer free.

The articles prompted her to check if the test was available through her gynecologist. Though her gynecologist used the test, it was more expensive than a pap smear, and her managed care plan paid only part of the cost. Because a past pap smear was "iffy" and one of her sisters had been treated for cervical cancer, she decided to pay $50 herself for the test. Her tests came back positive.

Your Personal Rx
If you have a chronic condition, like asthma or diabetes, subscribe to the national organization's newsletters, which often offer a rich supply of information on treatments and discoveries. The subscription is usually included in the organization membership. Most physicians we talked to recommended them for keeping current.

"Without the articles, I probably wouldn't have asked," she said. "I don't know for sure that the pap smear would have come back different than the new test, but I feel more secure that I got a better test. If I change plans, I'll ask more questions about the types of tests they pay for."

Newsletters, many affiliated with national medical centers or med schools, are also a big health business. Sometimes they deliver cutting-edge information, national trends, and good consumer information.

CD-ROMs can also be great visual teachers if your computer is fast enough to display the graphics. Though many CD-ROMs are geared toward anatomy, some are useful references for general family and pediatric care. The product line is expanding, though, to be more disease-specific. And a number of the CDs have links to useful sites on the Internet, lessening the chances of your $35–$50 investment becoming outdated too soon.

Treasures in the Public Library

Your health care bookshelf need not be confined to your home. Even the smallest public libraries have a limited supply of useful references.

The Big Books: Basic References

Most libraries have big reference books that are the standards in the field and comprehensive in scope. If you have a specific condition, or your curiosity has been piqued, the following titles are usually available no matter where you are:

➤ *Gray's Anatomy*, the grandaddy of medical references, is the classic text on human anatomy.

➤ The *Physician's Desk Reference* (published by Medical Economics) publishes versions on both prescription and over-the-counter drug products and preparations. They provide information on indications, interactions, side effects, and the danger of use during pregnancy.

Renowned medical centers such as Mount Sinai, Mayo Clinic, and Columbia University also publish home health guides most likely found in public libraries. You may also find the *Journal of the American Medical Association* (JAMA) or the *New England Journal of Medicine* (NEJM).

Public libraries are also the repository of government information. They have lots of publications from government agencies, including the U.S. Department of Health and Human Services, the National Institutes of Health, and many state agencies that deal with health issues. There is a wealth of information here, from how to get to health benefits for which you are entitled, to how to manage disabilities.

The New Librarian

Your local librarian is not there just to monitor noise levels or make sure your son doesn't hit the adult books too early. This is the age of the New Librarian, the information manager who can introduce you to the vast world of medical information. He can also help you structure and focus your search.

One of the outstanding services of the public library is providing access to the Internet. Many are investing in computer lines and equipment to better help them fulfill their mission: to provide knowledge tools to the public. Even without Internet access, most libraries are wired to access large databases of magazine indexes and regional, state, and university libraries. All this can be daunting for a first-time user, but the librarian can help you find your way. Remember, they are trained to assist the public, so don't be afraid to ask.

> **Your Personal Rx**
> A good way to "preview" books you may want to buy for your own home health bookshelf is to check out the ones in your library and see if they fit your needs. Libraries across the country are adding to their health sections because of consumer demand. Books and videos on everything from living with diabetes to healthy cooking to allergies can be found in the public library.

> **House Call**
> Public libraries answer an estimated 50 million health reference questions each year, and medical and other specialty libraries answer millions more, according to the U.S. Department of Health and Human Services.

The Internet: Surfers Beware

Your health care bookshelf may not even look like a shelf or a book. The Internet is key to accessing a wide variety of health care information, from chat groups of fellow migraine sufferers to the National Institutes of Health's online medical library.

For anyone with a chronic illness or disease, the Internet is essential. You have to be your own advocate, and one of the ways to do that successfully is by having up-to-date information. One of the problems of the Internet is that you use much of it at your own risk. Anybody can post so-called medical information on the Web, and sometimes it seems everyone who has snake oil to sell or an axe to grind has created a site. If you want to be as certain as possible of the accuracy of everything you read, stay with the government or established sources, like the New England Journal of Medicine Online or Mayo Online. If you can weigh the accuracy of the information, or you want to gather information and explore the accuracy later, there are almost unlimited resources on the Internet.

Government Megasites

Healthfinder (**http://www.healthfinder.gov**), which premiered in April 1997, is the federal government's collection of useful and responsible health and medical sites. The federal site covers a range of government agencies, nonprofits, support groups, and others. It's an Internet clearinghouse of sorts, put together to counter the enormous amount of misleading and wrong health information pervading the Internet. It's links to other government sites and a number of medical and health science libraries can save you valuable time.

Some other useful federal government sites (see the tearout card at the front of the book for all Website addresses):

➤ If you are traveling, the Centers for Disease Control offers publications online that cover infectious diseases and precautions. Their travel health information even has a clickable travel map with up-to-date immunization and travel precautions based on geographic area.

➤ The federal government also has Websites with up-to-the-minute information on specific diseases. The National Cancer Institute's CancerNet gives you access to medical libraries, treatment guidelines, clinical trials, pain management information, and much, much more. It gets approximately 1.5 million "hits" (visits) per month.

➤ Three cheers for Grateful Med. Grateful Med is the online National Library of Medicine. A bimonthly newsletter provides loads of new ideas on how to access this unparalleled resource. Check their site for details.

Many state-sponsored sites provide good medical information, but their strength is in providing information on their own state departments, including insurance commissioners, medical boards, and public health departments. The quality varies greatly. Many, however, give you directories of who to call and what to do if you have a complaint about doctors or health plans.

How Big Is the World Wide Web?

It is sooooo big. Approximately 10,000 sites on the Web contain medical consumer health information.

Above we've described the government Websites. University research centers also weigh in and are often tied to the government sites. Other sites are commercial sites set up by companies to sell and provide information on their products. That doesn't mean the information is untrue; it just can't be awarded a medal for being bias-free. Others are set up by individuals. Such a site can be the premier site on a particular topic, or it can be a wild harangue.

So what's a body to do? Evaluate Websites the same way you do books or magazines with medical information: Look at the credentials. Is the author and/or site affiliated with a well-known institution? Is it kept current, or was the last update six months ago (that's a lifetime on the Net). You can also check reviews in newspapers and family computing magazines for their take on whether the information in the site is reliable and beneficial.

You're Not Alone: Forums and Discussion Groups

One of the biggest breakthroughs of the Internet is the ability to tap into discussion groups with participants from around the world. There are thousands of discussion groups for parents, who can discuss the mundane (like parental fatigue syndrome) to the more serious (like cystic fibrosis). There are several managed care discussion groups, and it is often a topic in many other medical forums.

Online services host countless forums on health and often feature experts to take your questions. Chat groups, which are real-time discussions, are available on almost any health condition you can name. Some are moderated, which provides a cursory screening and tries to keep the "netiquette" civil. There is no screen for reliability, however.

Screen them the way you screen any discussion, whether at the grocery store check-out or at a support group meeting. Use your best judgment and follow up on information you may want to act upon with some research.

The Least You Need to Know

> ➤ Protect yourself with knowledge. Managed care plans expect health-literate members. You need to know how to find medical information if you want to succeed as your own (or a loved one's) advocate.

> ➤ Invest in a few health books for your home. Make sure they are easy to read and everyone who may have to use them knows where they are.

Your Personal Rx
The Web is a great place to find out whether the National Committee on Quality Assurance has accredited your health care plan or to compare health plans in your area. The California Business Group on Health has excellent information on California plans (see Appendix B for addresses). Many managed care plans have their own sites, with the quality ranging from somewhat helpful to as useful as your member handbook.

Your Personal Rx
Discussion groups are located on the Usenet, and you can often find references to them in Websites. Sometimes chat groups can be part of some Websites. Sometimes online services such as America Online have announcements for specially scheduled chats. You can find discussion groups by using search engines such as Dejanews (www.dejanews.com), which search discussion groups by using keyword searches just like you use for Websites.

➤ Libraries can be your best resource. You can preview books, check out references and journals, and use databases and the Internet to get your answers.

➤ Medical information is no longer behind the heavy doors of research institutes but on the Internet on your computer screen right there in your family room. But knowing what is reliable and what is unreliable can be tricky: Look at who is providing the information and check out their credentials.

Part 2
Choosing (and Paying for) Your Coverage

What's smaller than a mortgage payment and bigger than most car payments? Give up? It's what you (and your employer, if you're lucky) pay for your health care coverage, month after (hopefully uneventful) month.

With all this money at stake, you'd think they'd let you test-drive health plans, wouldn't you? Well, they don't. Most of us have one shot at choosing a plan, at least until open season comes along at work or we change jobs, and no chance to check out the "feel" of the available options. It's as if you had to buy a car without seeing how it accelerates on the highway or whether your skis will fit in the roof rack—and little prospect of trading it in any time soon.

But wait! Don't throw up your hands in despair and start hunting for the TV Guide. Help is as near as the next page! In this section, we talk about comparing the cost, coverage, and quality features of the plans available to you. We show you the special ways to get into the system when you change jobs, start your own business, or pass important life milestones such as getting married, having a baby, getting divorced, then getting married again, and retiring. We also talk about managed care in rural areas and in Medicaid. We don't care who you are; we've got you covered.

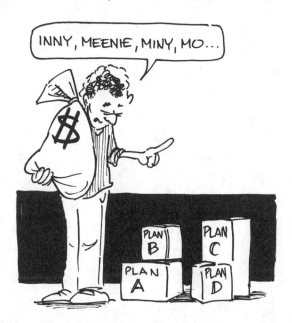

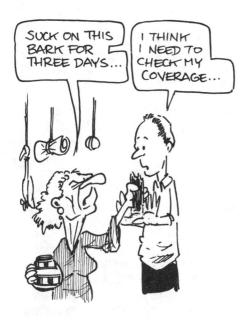

Chapter 5

More Than a Paycheck: Choosing Health Care Coverage Through Your Job

> **In This Chapter**
>
> ➤ Untangling the web of health care plans
>
> ➤ Considering a plan's provisions
>
> ➤ Calculating the costs
>
> ➤ Putting away rainy day dollars

Most people get health care coverage from their employer or that of a spouse or parent. So, if you change jobs 10 times during your life, you'll encounter 10 different health plans.

Or not. Maybe your first employer changed health plans five times during the 10 years you were there. Maybe four of your employers gave you the option of choosing your favorite health plan, though you could have chosen another. And for your remaining six employers, you had to choose among four plans each time you changed jobs.

Congrats! You had the not-so-rare opportunity to wade through the brochures, videos, and Websites of 52 health care plans.

In this chapter we begin to show you how to compare plans (for more on this, see Chapter 6). If you don't have a choice of your health plan, you can skip much of this chapter for now. Read it again if you change jobs, if your employer changes plans, or if you have questions about what your plan covers.

So Many Choices...

We love our freedom to choose. Over half of all private-sector employees with employer-based health care coverage can choose from among plans, and many can choose from among three or more.

The odds of having choices may depend on where you live or work. Urban residents generally have more choices than residents of small communities or rural areas. Those working for smaller firms may also have more health plan choices than in the past; although small firms are still the least likely to offer their employees coverage, let alone a choice. They are usually lucky to be able to offer health coverage at all. Now, with the emergence of local purchasing coalitions that are open to many different employers, even some small firms offer their employees a choice of plans. On the other hand, some larger employers are narrowing the range of choices they offer their employees, typically by excluding traditional *fee-for-service* plans.

Before you begin to decide among your health care plan options, you need to understand the basic structure of the plans available to you. If you've read Chapter 1, you should be able to tell the difference between the managed care and fee-for-service plans. You have to know the difference. If you can't distinguish between the two, it will lead to costly and potentially harmful mistakes. If you aren't sure, go back to Chapter 1 or call your employee benefits office before reading further.

After you've sorted out the managed health care plans from the fee-for-service plans, you also need to consider the following:

➤ Plan provisions (what's in a plan)

➤ Cost

➤ Quality

➤ Your own health care needs

➤ The location of providers or facilities you may be required or encouraged to use

The rest of this chapter explains how to evaluate the plan provisions and cost. See Chapter 6 for information on assessing a plan's quality.

What's in a Plan: Understanding What Your Plan Will Cover

When you choose your health care plan, consider the plan's provisions, or what the plan includes. Think about these three things:

➤ What it covers or *covered services*

➤ What it doesn't cover or its *exclusions*

➤ What it covers, to a point, also called its *limitations*

Covered Services

Make sure the plan you are considering covers the care you and your family need. Bear in mind that everything in health care coverage depends both on how the plan is written and on the patient's individual medical circumstances. For your plan to pay *anything*, the services you receive must be *covered* and *medically necessary*. The amount the plan pays, from nothing to the full amount, will depend on its provisions.

The services your plan covers are usually defined in a section of your plan booklet entitled "General Information" or "Covered Services." Look also for a "Glossary" or another definitions section for important information.

You can divide covered services into three groups:

➤ Those that all plans offer

➤ Those that most plans offer

➤ Those that some plans offer

Here are the basic services covered by almost all health plans:

➤ Hospital room and board

➤ Inpatient and outpatient surgery

➤ Inpatient and office physician visits

➤ Services of nurses and sometimes licensed practical nurses

➤ Diagnostic and X-ray laboratory tests

Healthspeak
Covered services are the medically necessary treatments your plan undertakes to pay for, at least in part. *Medically necessary* treatments are those that are appropriate for the diagnosis, care, or treatment of the injury or condition involved. Standards of medical necessity can differ among plans. If a service is not medically necessary, the plan won't pay for it.

Caution
It is common for plans to limit their coverage to care provided by legally qualified physicians and other health care professionals. If your doctor loses his license to practice medicine, your plan will not pay for his services.

Ambulance services (when medically necessary) and rentals of medical equipment that may be necessary for therapy or for home care (such as hospital beds or wheelchairs) are also typically covered.

After this point, plans become a little pickier in terms of what they will do for you. Most, but not all, plans cover *extended care, home health care, hospice care,* and *inpatient* and *outpatient* mental health and *alcohol and substance abuse treatment. Extended care* facilities provide skilled nursing care, rehabilitation, and convalescent services to patients requiring less intensive treatment than a hospital provides. *Home health care* is skilled nursing and related care supplied to a patient at home, usually after being hospitalized. Hospice care is given to terminally ill patients—generally those with six months or less to live—

and emphasizes meeting emotional needs and coping with pain. Care may be given in the patient's home or in a separate facility. Inpatient alcohol and substance abuse treatments focus on detoxification and rehabilitation. Detoxification is the use of medication and other methods under medical supervision to reduce or eliminate the effects of alcohol or substance abuse. Rehabilitation is designed to change patients' behaviors once they are free of acute physical and mental complications. Rehabilitation may be in the hospital or not. Most plans cover mental health and substance abuse treatment differently from treatments for other conditions.

Nearly all HMOs also cover preventive care (see Chapter 12). Preventive care includes physical examinations, well-baby care, and immunization and inoculations. Nearly all HMOs also cover hearing care, though the coverage may not extend beyond hearing examinations (see Chapter 8 for special provisions for seniors in Medicare HMOs). Hearing exams are important for the elderly, who are more likely to suffer hearing impairments, but should also be a part of routine preventive care for children.

Most non-HMO plans do not cover preventive care, but enough do that you should certainly check. Most plans do not cover birthing center services, but non-HMO plans are more likely to do so than HMOs.

Dental or vision care may be offered as part of a comprehensive medical plan or as separate plans that can be chosen in addition to any medical plan. You may have to pay separately for your coverage, or you may incur costs only if you use services. You may receive discounts or benefits only if you use preferred providers, or you may be reimbursed for usual and customary charges regardless of the provider you select.

Procedures costing over a certain amount may be subject to advance authorization to be covered. Check your plan documents or ask your plan's member services department before you commit yourself.

Exclusions, Limitations, and Pre-Existing Conditions

Plan *exclusions* and *limitations* are as important as covered services. Look for these in your plan booklet or descriptive material under a heading such as "General Exclusions and Limitations." Once you are a member, you may have to read both the plan's basic document and updates or amendments.

Healthspeak
Exclusions are medical coverages, services, or conditions for which a particular health care plan or policy will not provide or pay. Plan *limitations* tell you when a covered treatment isn't covered.

Plans issue updates when their coverage changes (rather than revising their whole plan description) in part to highlight for you what has changed. Otherwise, revisions could be buried in material you thought you already understood. Even in cases where the "update" is several years old, you may have to wade through several documents to get the whole picture.

Among the most common exclusions and limitations in non-HMO plans are those for *pre-existing conditions*. HMO plans can't impose such conditions because they offer you comprehensive care.

You've probably heard the horror stories of children with heart conditions unable to get the care they need or adults with cancer left out in the cold when a spouse changes plans. These people often get into trouble because of pre-existing condition limitations. A new federal law may ease the burden for many of these people and their families (see Chapter 7 for a full discussion).

Once you've unearthed the general exclusions and limitations, read on. Plans often list 30 or more separate exclusions and limitations, many of which are related to each other. You may be in for some surprises, so read your documents carefully. Here is a cross section of common exclusions and limitations:

> **Healthspeak**
> A *pre-existing condition*—mental or physical—is one that began before the plan member became covered under a particular plan. The amount of time before something is no longer considered "pre-existing" varies greatly. Some plans limit the amount they will pay for treating such a condition—or won't cover it at all—for a period of time.

➤ Many plans do not cover pregnancies and related care until the employee or covered dependent has been enrolled in the plan for at least 10 months. After 1998, most will no longer be able to do this (more on this in Chapter 7).

➤ Most won't pay for services for conception by artificial means, but some plans will pay for artificial insemination. Treatment for a medical problem that leads to infertility should be covered under most plans.

➤ Most plans won't pay for reversing voluntary sterilization procedures, such as vasectomies or tubal ligations.

➤ Oral contraceptive pills are typically included in a plan's prescription drug coverage, but diaphragms, intrauterine devices (IUDs), and other contraceptive drugs may not be covered.

➤ Elective abortions are often excluded, but those considered medically necessary may be covered.

➤ Because people donate blood, it's free, right? WRONG! Blood *is* free, but it has to be processed to be used by a patient. These processing costs can be substantial, and are often excluded from coverage.

➤ Gender reassignment (sex change) treatments or surgeries will most likely not be covered, but surgeries to correct congenital defects will.

➤ Cosmetic surgery is typically not covered, but such surgery necessitated by an injury, disease, or birth defect is generally covered. Some plans do not cover breast reconstruction after mastectomy.

➤ Many plans exclude various types of orthodontic treatments.

➤ Experimental or investigational treatments are commonly excluded from coverage. However, both plans and medical experts may often differ in what they consider experimental or investigational (see Chapter 18 for more on experimental and investigational treatments).

➤ If the plan covers nonexperimental organ transplants, it may restrict the type of transplant covered, referrals for such treatment, or both. Don't expect coverage for transplants using nonhuman organs.

➤ Patients with disabilities related to military service can be required to obtain care at a Veterans Administration facility.

➤ Treatment for on-the-job injuries covered by workers' compensation, auto insurance, or similar laws is often excluded. You can usually obtain the care and provide the information about the other coverage to your plan to allow it to recover.

➤ Marriage and relationship therapy may be excluded even in plans that cover mental health care.

➤ Mental health services ordered by a court may not be covered unless they are medically necessary.

Out of Your Pocket

Healthspeak
Provider discounts are reduced rates doctors, hospitals, and other health care professionals or facilities agree to accept when they enroll in a health plan's network.

Healthspeak
A *cafeteria* plan allows employees to choose benefits from a number of different options, including pensions and savings, a health plan, other insurance, and time off. A *flexible spending account* allows employees to set aside pretax earnings to pay for benefits or expenses that are not paid by their insurance or benefit plans. A flexible spending account may be free-standing or part of a cafeteria plan.

Once you decide which plans cover the services and treatments important to you, you are ready to look at plan costs. We favor "value buying" or finding the best combination of cost and value to suit your needs. The more restrictive the plan on the choice of doctors, hospitals, and such, the less it should cost.

So what's your bottom-line cost? What you pay out-of-pocket will depend on the interaction of the plan's various cost provisions: copayments or coinsurance, deductibles, annual limits, and *provider discounts*. Add in the differences among plans in your share of premiums, what the plan covers, how much it pays for what it covers, your health and that of your family, and your approach to using health care. Here are the major factors that will influence your bottom line.

Employee Contributions: You Help Pay for Coverage

Most employers who offer health care coverage pay for at least part of its cost, and some pay for all of it. But most employees have to chip in something.

Look at your paycheck. What is the deduction for health care coverage? About half of all employees have to contribute something, and most have to pay something toward family coverage. There can be certain tax benefits that may offset your yearly cost. If your employer offers *a flexible spending account* or a *cafeteria* plan, you may be able to pay your share of the premium on a tax-exempt basis. Check with your human resources department or tax preparer for details.

Deductibles: You Pay First

Nearly all fee-for-service plans and the majority of PPO plans impose *deductibles*. Some plans apply a single deductible—typically around $200 for individuals and two to three times that for families—to all services covered under the plan. Others apply separate deductibles to specific categories of expenses. For instance, you can be charged a separate deductible for each hospital admission. PPOs that require you to pay a deductible often offer lower deductibles if you stick to network providers. An advantage of HMOs is that they typically do not have deductibles.

Employers and insurance companies use deductibles in their plans for several reasons. People spend more when someone else is paying the bill than when they do. A deductible makes people think twice about getting care for a minor problem, especially if it might go away by itself. In PPO and POS plans, a deductible can serve as an incentive for you to use providers the plan has selected if in-network care is subject to a lower or no deductible. A deductible also frees plans from having to write and mail lots of small checks.

Usually, the higher the deductible, the lower the premiums both for the employer and the employee. But be careful about enrolling in a high deductible plan just for the savings. Deductibles can be as high as $1,000 for individual coverage. These plans are sometimes called "catastrophic" plans, because they only start paying once you have incurred significant medical expenses in a given year. Don't put such a plan on your list unless:

Healthspeak
A *deductible* is the amount of covered expenses that an individual must pay before any charges are paid by the medical care plan.

Your Personal Rx
Deductibles may lead to the "shoebox effect." Many people will keep small medical bills in a shoebox until they accumulate enough to make it worth filing a claim form—and then lose the box or forget to file! If you have to file, do it as soon as possible. You could lose money if you miss deadlines or lose your records.

➤ The plan imposes no deductible, or a lower one, if you use doctors, hospitals, and others in its network.

➤ Your spouse or other household member has a comprehensive health care coverage plan that gives you secondary coverage.

➤ You are willing and able to set aside money—in a regular savings account or in a tax-preferred flexible spending account—to pay for care until your deductible is met.

The high deductible can also discourage you from obtaining even preventive or urgent care that you *should* have.

Copayments and Coinsurance: You Pay Again

Healthspeak
Copayments are fixed-dollar payments the patient makes per doctor visit or per prescription filled. For example, many HMOs and PPOs impose a copayment (sometimes called a "copay") of $5 or $10 for an in-network physician visit. Under *coinsurance,* you and the plan each pay a share of the provider's charges.

Copayments and *coinsurance* sound alike and are often used interchangeably, but they are not the same thing. They have different consequences to your health care costs. Copayments for health care or prescription drugs are set without regard to the provider's usual charges. Coinsurance, on the other hand, is a percentage of the provider's charges that you are required to pay.

Depending on the type of plan you choose, your coinsurance rate may be different if you use in-network providers (often 10 percent) than if you go outside the network (often 30 percent). Your out-of-pocket costs for using an out-of-network provider will depend on how much the provider usually charges. This gives you an incentive to shop around or use providers in your network.

Annual Limits

If a major illness or injury strikes you or your family, how much can you afford to pay? How much does your health plan say it will pay? Your plan may have one or more annual limits on the amount you are expected to spend, the amount the plan will spend for you, or both. Limits on what the plan will pay are common in non-HMO plans. Limits on what you are expected to pay occur in all types of plans.

Caution
If you have a large family or a chronic health condition, take a close look at copays and coinsurance. Some plans don't require the member to spend anything other than the premium. In other plans, you pay the regular coinsurance or copayment no matter how much you have already spent in a given year.

Most plans limit the amount you must pay in a given year. Your spending is counted toward this limit once your plan deductible has been met. A typical limit is $1,000 to $2,000 under individual coverage and about twice that under family coverage; then the plan will pay 100 percent of your health care costs. If you are enrolled in an HMO plan that charges copayments, you may not be required to make any more such payments once your total spending exceeds two times your annual premium. The maximum out-of-pocket costs to the consumer are called the plan's stop-loss provisions.

Most people in non-HMO plans also have a limit on the benefits their plan will pay out during their lifetime. For most people in plans with benefit maximums, the limit is at least $500,000, but it really varies: Some are as high as a million and some as low as $25,000. Even with a high lifetime limit, a premature baby, chronic mental illness, or severe head injury can exhaust those benefits. But many plans have no lifetime limits.

Getting to the Bottom Line

We developed a simple worksheet you can use to check how all these factors work together and compare the costs. To use it, pick two plans that appeal to you based on quality, structure, convenience, or other criteria. (If you don't want to be limited to two plans, photocopy the worksheet and complete it for as many as you like!)

Use your own (or your family's) experience (or best "guesstimate") last year. If you were the picture of health, put in a "what if" cost item, such as outpatient knee surgery. Fill in the costs based on your experience and the plans you are considering. You will quickly know which plan will cost you or you and your family the least over the coming year. What are you willing to give up to save money? Completing the worksheet will allow you to gauge how much various plan features are worth to you.

House Call

You may have coverage under more than one plan. Maybe you and your husband are covered under each other's plan, or your college student has a school policy in addition to your family coverage. To save money, let your doctors and hospitals know about all your coverage. Your plans will coordinate their payments so that your total benefits do not exceed your allowable medical expenses.

We have calculated out-of-pocket costs for a hypothetical member in the column marked "Example." Here's how to use the worksheet:

➤ Item #1: Multiply the amount your employer deducts from each paycheck by the number of paychecks you receive per year. Enter 0 (zero) here if the coverage is provided to you at no cost.

➤ Item # 2: Take your usual number of doctor's visits per year and multiply by your plan's copayment (our example assumes you pay $10 per visit). If the plans use coinsurance, multiply that rate (say, 30 percent or .30) by the provider's usual charges (say, $100 per visit). Don't forget to include annual preventive care appointments, kids' check-ups, and the occasional flu or ear infection. If any of the plans you are comparing impose a deductible, count 100 percent of your doctor visits or other medical costs for those plans until the deductible is met.

➤ Item #3: Do the same thing for prescriptions that you did in #2. Multiply the number of prescriptions you have filled during a year by the plan's copayment, or by your coinsurance rate times the retail price, as applicable. Be sure to consider each prescription refill separately.

➤ Item #4: Insert one major health care expense here, more if you need a lot of health care. If you have some real expenses from a previous year, say, for knee surgery, plug them in here. If you used a plan with a network of providers who offer discounts to its members, just plug in your share of the costs here. Our example assumes that we used a network provider. Typically discounted fees are 10 to 20 percent below the usual rates.

➤ Item #5: List your out-of-pocket costs under your plan options. Various plans may exclude either services you want or may not fully cover providers you want. Our example assumes that none of the itemized services are covered. Don't list expenses that none of the plans available to you cover or discount. They will be your expenses no matter what you chose.

Your Personal Plan Comparison Worksheet

Item #	Cost Item	Example	Plan 1	Plan 2
1	Your share of premiums (if monthly, × 12)	$100 × 12 = $1,200		
2	Usual # of doctor visits × copayment	6 × $10 = $60		
3	# of prescriptions per year × copayment (or coinsurance rate × usual and customary charges)	10 × $5 = $50		
4	1 episode of outpatient surgery	$1,000 × .10 = $100		
5	Cost of noncovered services (# of visits × full charge) Chiropractor Nutritionist for food allergy follow-up Marriage counseling Add other expenses (for example, glasses, hearing aids)	6 × $35 = $210 3 × $55 = $165 6 × $90 = $540 $200		
6	Gross health care costs − $200 tax savings from establishing flexible spending account for non-covered medical expenses Net health care costs	$1,325 −199 $1,126		

➤ Item #6: Consider the tax factor. If your employer allows you to make pretax contributions to a flexible spending amount, your out-of-pocket costs are reduced by the amount of taxes you save on such contributions. In our example, we have assumed that the person put the entire amount of expected out-of-pocket costs ($1,325) into a flexible spending account. The tax savings would be $199 (0.15 × $1,325, rounded to the nearest dollar). Your net health care costs are your total out-of-pocket outlays, minus your tax savings, if any.

Caution
When considering a flexible spending account, remember that you will lose any money you don't use by the end of the plan year. So don't put in a large amount unless you expect to need it.

Your Rainy Day Fund

If you can, include at least one fee-for-service plan in your plan comparison, even if you are pretty sure a managed care plan is what you want. This way, you will know how much managed care is saving you. Your trade-off is some of your freedom of health care choice for lower costs.

Take these cost savings and...save them!

Someday, you may urgently want care that the plan is unwilling to pay for—and you want it in a hurry. If you put these savings aside—and don't touch them—you may be able to pay for that test or minor surgery yourself (more on this in Chapters 16, 17, 18, and 23).

Caution
Don't put your rainy day fund into your employer's flexible spending account or cafeteria plan. Your rainy day fund should be long-term, "quiet" money.

The Least You Need to Know

➤ Health care plans don't all cover the same medical services and treatments and may not pay the entire cost of those they do cover.

➤ Whether a service or treatment is covered or excluded under your plan depends on how the plan documents are worded. The plan may specifically exclude them, exclude them under certain circumstances, or omit them from a list of covered services.

➤ Even if the services are covered, you may not be able to get them through the plan if your doctor and/or the plan does not consider them to be medically necessary. Your doctor may be helpful in explaining your case to your plan.

➤ Your out-of-pocket health care costs will generally depend both on how much health care you use and on how you use it.

Chapter 6

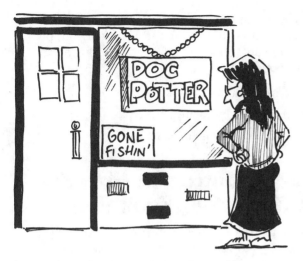

Getting the Most for Your Money: Evaluating Plan Quality

In This Chapter

➤ Outcomes data: Can your plan pass the math?

➤ How to check on your plan's "good care" commitment

➤ How to read their report cards

➤ Picking the plan that's right for you

Most people wouldn't buy a car without checking its performance-related features like repair rates, crash test results, and car reviews. You talk to friends and family members who own, have owned, or knew somebody who owned the same model.

You (and your employer, if you're lucky) probably spend more each month on your health insurance than you do on your car payment. And that's year in, year out—it never gets paid off!

Just as all cars are not the same, neither are all health care plans. Government regulation generally ensures that health plans, doctors, labs, and hospitals meet certain minimal standards (more on this in Chapter 25). But not all licensed or otherwise accredited plans and providers are of equal quality. Some are better than others at handling basic medical care, while others are better equipped to handle rare, exceptional cases.

Your managed care plan can be your port in a storm or your worst nightmare. A good plan can increase the chances you will receive the preventive care you need to stay well. Should you fall sick, a good plan increases the chances you will experience a full and uneventful recovery. A bad plan does just the opposite.

Caution
Notice we used the word "minimal" when describing government standards. Much of government regulation has to do with financial stability, not quality of care, and medical boards and state regulators have been under attack for slow reaction to reports of dangerous doctors. Though both federal and state governments are working on providing information on health care quality, actual regulation is limited.

Healthspeak
Health care *outcomes* measure the impact of the health care system— doctor visits, hospital stays, surgeries—on specific measures of patients' health. Such measures include survival rates and complication rates after various surgeries.

Fortunately, you can find out a lot about your health. This chapter tells you how to evaluate the quality of your plan or the plans you are thinking of joining, focusing on the following important measures:

➤ Health care *outcomes*

➤ Health care use by their members

➤ How satisfied their members are

Evaluating Outcomes: How the Plan Affects Your Health

Managed care plans love to use percentages, scores, ratios, charts, and graphs to show that they offer great care. Anyone who deals with health care statistics knows how "creative" playing with those numbers can be. So ask questions, do your best in interpreting their stats, and simply ask yourself, "Can this plan pass the math?"

One of the ways to compare plan quality is to compare the plans' impact on their members' health outcomes. Outcomes are usually expressed as percentages, sometimes of members in the plan, sometimes of a specific sector of their members (for example, pregnancies in the plan). Outcomes data you most likely will see are:

➤ Babies with low birth weights

➤ Patients who acquire infections while in the hospital

➤ Patients experiencing other post-surgery complications

➤ Heart disease and stroke patients who die while in the hospital

➤ Patients with high blood pressure who achieve normal blood pressure after one year of treatment

Some outcomes measures are clearly good results, so a higher score is better. For example, a large proportion of patients with high blood pressure under control is good, while a lower proportion is not as good. Other outcomes measures are clearly "bad," so look for a plan with lower percentages in those areas. For example, plans would want to keep their scores on the first four measures listed above as low as possible.

A plan's score on a particular measure doesn't give you the full picture. You also need information on how well other plans do. We return to this issue later in this chapter in the discussion of plan "report cards."

Outcomes measures are useful when you decide which plan to choose, because a plan that does well with certain groups of patients is likely to give good care to most of its members. For example, if more people die after heart attacks, or more women with breast cancer die within five years of their diagnosis in the hypothetical PANES Plan than in the equally hypothetical ACHES Plan, we can say that the ACHES Plan takes "better" care of its members' health.

Outcomes measures, however, are relatively new and can be difficult to interpret, even by our hero, the Informed Consumer. Many conditions and treatments do not yet have outcomes measures. Even if there are measures, it is difficult to adjust them to reflect what the membership of the plan looks like. For example, if a plan's members are generally older than those in another plan, their outcomes are likely to be worse.

House Call

Many plans may not publish their outcomes data, even when available, because they serve a less-healthy population. Their reported outcomes may be poor because their members are sicker or older, not because they provide poor care. Sometimes outcomes data are adjusted for differences in the characteristics of plan members, but these adjustments are difficult and controversial.

You can get outcomes data from the plans when the marketing folks meet with you during open enrollment (the time when you are able to switch plans). Sometimes business groups and coalitions or local health organizations will use such data in information sheets. Some groups publish books about choosing plans in large metropolitan areas; they will list outcomes data.

So, does your plan pass the math? It may be hard to tell. If you have a particular concern, like a chronic disease, pregnancy, or possible surgery, ask if your plan representative has outcomes data for it. Use it, but don't be blinded by the numbers. Outcomes research has a long way to go.

Getting the Care You Need (and No More)

Since measuring the *results* of health care has its limitations, you may also want to look at how the plan *delivers* the care in the first place. This includes:

➤ Whether it's easy or hard to get care

➤ How hard the plan is likely to work to keep you healthy

➤ How much the plan does to (or for, depending on your perspective) its members

Your Personal Rx

A great list of doctors doesn't get you great care if they aren't accepting new patients from your plan. If you are joining a new plan, call the doctor and ask if he is accepting new patients from your plan. Sometimes the plan's directory will have an asterisk (*) next to the names of doctors who are in your plan but are no longer accepting new patients.

The Doctor is In (But Will She See You)?

Most of us head for the doctor's office only when we need to (or are afraid we need to). While waiting in a long line for a first-run movie can add to your excitement and anticipation, waiting days for an appointment and hours to be seen does not.

Ask about where the plan's doctors and hospitals are located and how many doctors are seeing new patients. A great list of doctors means nothing to you if the doctors are always booked way ahead. You should also ask how long you will typically have to wait for an appointment and at the doctor's office. Also ask what they do for after-hours, urgent, and emergency care (more on emergency care in Chapter 14). The plan should be able to provide this information.

Getting Preventive Care

You know all those healthy people in the marketing brochures? Managed care plans use them to convince you that they have great preventive care. Would you join a plan where everyone looked sick?

Preventive care is very important; the plan should be working to keep you healthy (for more on preventive care, see Chapter 12). Information on how well a plan delivers preventive care usually shows what percentage (they love percentages) of certain members received specific types of preventive care. Some examples include:

➤ Children immunized

➤ Adults whose cholesterol has been screened

➤ Women who have received mammograms or have been screened for cervical cancer

➤ Pregnant women who received prenatal care in the first trimester

➤ Diabetics receiving a retinal exam

➤ Children with asthma who are hospitalized

In the preceding list, higher scores are better on all the items except for pediatric asthma hospitalization rates; good preventive care means the child stays out of the hospital.

It doesn't matter whether these are conditions that affect you now or that you ever expect to be concerned about. If the plan is checking up on people with these conditions, it is probably also checking up on the conditions that could affect you.

Procedure Rates

Preventive care, of course, doesn't prevent everything. You also need to know what the plan does when you need more. Look at how often the plan performs some procedures that are widely believed to be overused:

➤ Gall-bladder removal

➤ Prostate surgery

➤ Hysterectomy

➤ Deliveries by Caesarean section

Some differences on these measures among plans can be expected based on what their membership looks like. For example, a plan serving an area with a lot of retirees may perform fewer Cesarean sections and more gall-bladder removals (but see the discussion on interpreting plan report cards in the section titled "Report Cards" later in this chapter).

Consumer Satisfaction

Is a happy consumer a healthy consumer? Not always. You may leave your doctor's office grumpy if you haven't gotten an antibiotic for your sniffles, even though you don't need—and your sniffles wouldn't respond to—antibiotics. On the other hand, your Aunt Jan who is on six medications may feel her doctor is vigilant, even though she needs only one prescription.

Your Personal Rx
Be wary of plans that perform a lot—or very few—of the procedures listed here. Plans may offer a lot of surgery because they think it will make their members happy, not because the members need it. On the other hand, plans that do much less than their competition may be denying surgery to some people who do need it. Look for a balance.

Plans that are seeking (or working to keep) accreditation generally have to have procedures in place for measuring consumer satisfaction (more on this in Chapter 25). Some of the consumer satisfaction measures you may see in plan brochures include:

➤ Waiting times (for appointments and in doctors' offices)

➤ Choice and convenience of physicians

➤ Ratings of personal treatment by the doctor or other provider, including their communication skills and personal interest in you and your condition

➤ How well and efficiently the plan deals with problems or complaints

➤ Whether the respondent would recommend the doctor, hospital, or plan to their family or friends

➤ The percentage of respondents renewing their plan membership

These can be useful for an overall sense of how well the plan is run and how oriented it is to serving its members. But remember: The plans themselves report this information, even to their own accrediting organizations, and very few plan reports are independently audited at the present time. Your best defense against selectively reported—let alone misreported—information is to take as broad a perspective on plan performance data as possible. In other words, read all the information you get as if your life depended on it!

Report Cards

Managed care plans, competing for your enrollment, are likely to show you what they call a "report card," or a summary of their ratings on aspects of plan performance. *HEDIS* is a widely used rating system that has become the HMO industry's standard for measuring quality. If possible, compare a plan's HEDIS data with similar data for all plans.

Healthspeak
The National Committee for Quality Assurance (NCQA)—an independent, not-for-profit organization formed by the HMO industry—developed a set of health care quality measures known as the Health Plan Employer Data and Information Set (*HEDIS*). *HEDIS* consists of statistics on health care delivered by plans, including preventive care and rates for certain surgical procedures.

Be warned that HEDIS data are reported by the plans themselves, and most are not audited by an impartial third party. This means that the information is a "best effort," but there is no 100 percent guarantee it is right. HEDIS data may also be difficult for individual consumers to use, at least without some guidance.

NCQA also publishes the averages of 17 HEDIS measurements (see the table below) and updates them regularly. The data give the national average score on each measure for the HMO plans participating in their survey. Participation is voluntary, so plans with good records may be more likely to participate.

National Averages for Selected HMO Quality Measures, 1997

Quality Indicator	National Average
Preventive care	
Children with required immunizations by age 2	78.6%
Adults age 40 to 64 screened for cholesterol	69.7%
Women age 52 to 64 with a mammogram in past two years	69.1%
Women age 21 to 64 with a Pap smear in past three years	73.7%
Women giving birth with prenatal care early in their pregnancy	87.5%
Patients hospitalized for depression with an outpatient visit within 30 days of discharge	76.9%
Diabetics with a retinal exam in the last calendar year	37.3%
Health care access	
Members who have seen a provider for care in the past three years:	
age 23–39	88.0%
age 40–64	88.9%
Quality of care	
Average maternity care hospital stay for women ages 15–34	2.01%

Quality Indicator	National Average
Caesarean section rate	19.6%
Patients readmitted within 365 days of discharge:	
Mental health	15.3%
Chemical dependency	14.1%
Quality of providers	
Percentage of physicians board certified:	
Primary care	79.6%
Specialists	82.9%

Source: National Committee on Quality Assurance Quality Compass (http://www.ncqa.org), March 19, 1997. Percents based on 250 plans.

Understanding the Scores

Seventeen measures is a lot of data to handle, so we divide them into four categories that you can use to compare plans.

In the "preventive care" category, the higher the plan's score, the better the plan is at reaching individuals in a given group of patients (pregnant women, diabetics, and so on).

"Health care access" measures how easy it is for plan members to get to certain health care providers. A higher score is "better." If a plan does not enroll enough physicians accepting new patients, new patients may face unacceptably long waits for appointments or needed care.

House Call

The number of available doctors can be a problem, particularly in areas with a large number of competing managed care plans. A doctor may belong to lots of plans but limit the number of patients he'll accept. Consumers should look at the proportion of participating physicians accepting new patients.

"Quality of care" measures the plan's performance for patients with selected conditions. Unlike measures of preventive care or health care access, a high score in this category is not always better. High Caesarean section rates or rates of re-admission among mental health and chemical dependency patients, for example, can indicate poor patient management by the plan.

Board certification of primary care doctors and specialists is another good measure of quality, shown in the table under "Quality of providers." Almost everyone we talked to told us that board certification is highly important when picking doctors and plans.

Ranking the Hospitals

Not every plan contracts with every hospital in your area, and, if you have lots of hospitals near you, knowing how good a hospital is can be very useful. The Center for the Study of Services, a consumer watchdog organization based in Washington, D.C., has a Website for this very purpose (see Appendix B). The Center's "Healthcheck" page plans to offer searchable online consumers' guides to hospitals, health plans, and physicians. As we wrote this book, only the guide to hospitals was available in an online edition. Print versions of the *Consumers' Guide to Hospitals and Health Plans* are available for purchase and at many libraries.

Who Says So?

Not too long ago, surveys and report cards asked questions like, "Are you ecstatically, sublimely, or very happy with your care?"

Your report would be "very happy," and the news services would report it.

With increased competition and more familiarity with managed care (and their marketing), ratings and reports are getting more realistic. Still, when you look at report cards for plans or hospitals, ask what group is represented in the ratings:

➤ Is it all the people served by the plan, anywhere? If so, the plan's performance in your locality could differ from that in other communities. There are local factors that come into play, such as physician and hospital availability.

➤ Is it all your employer's employees served by the plan? Many people pay the most attention to data based on their fellow employees' experience. But it might not be very useful to you if your employer has sites all over the country and the report card does not separate out ratings for your locality.

➤ Is it all the people served by the plan in your community? If you work for a small firm, this information may be as detailed as you will be able to get. Your firm alone may not be large enough for a valid survey.

In addition to materials prepared by your employer and/or the plans you are considering, you may also want to look at local and national publications:

➤ *Consumer Reports* is a national publication that conducts occasional surveys of managed care plan performance and consumer satisfaction.

➤ *Health Pages* is a magazine that focuses on cost and benefit comparisons of different local health plans.

➤ The Center for the Study of Services publishes guides to doctors, hospitals, and health plans.

Regional business coalitions and local chambers also have information. If you are a federal or state government employee or retiree, your local newspaper may publish lists of "best buys," or best benefits for the least money, around open enrollment time. See Chapter 4 for more information on how to find the books and other resources you need to do your homework on health care.

What's Right for You

This chapter gave you lots of advice on what data about quality are available to you. Use them with this caveat: You are an individual with a unique medical history and prospects. Your own circumstances and medical care style will help determine the type of plan that will serve you best.

The table printed below gives you a checklist of plan performance items to think about in picking a plan. We use the term "loose network" to refer to a PPO or POS plan that reimburses you for the cost of out-of-network providers, even if at a lower rate than if you seek care within the network. A "tight network" is an HMO or similar plan that restricts you to network providers to receive any reimbursement at all. Use this checklist together with your personal plan cost worksheet from Chapter 5 to narrow down your plan options to the one that will provide you with the best value for your money.

Health Care Coverage Options for You

Your situation	Your best option may be...
You have a chronic condition and want to be sure to be treated by a specialist.	Some tight networks, or a loose network without gatekeeper requirements; more on chronic conditions in Chapter 15.
The plans you have available don't do well with your condition.	A loose network; you may be able to get out-of-network referrals more easily.
Your plan options do not have the specialists or the hospitals you would like to use.	A loose network; again, referrals may be easier to get.
You prefer one-stop shopping for your health care needs.	A tight network; all of your needs will be met in one plan, possibly under one roof.
You have a pre-existing condition and have recently had time without health care coverage.	Either, depending on plan provisions, but see Chapter 7 for more on what happens when you change plans or lose your coverage.
You have a condition with no standard treatments available and would like to be able to explore promising new treatments.	A loose network; more on getting access to new treatments in Chapter 17.

The Least You Need to Know

➤ All health care plans, doctors, and hospitals are not alike. Some do a much better job, especially with selected health care conditions, than others.

➤ When evaluating health plan report cards, make sure you are given some standards for comparison.

➤ A plan you are considering should be able to tell you how easily you can get a doctor's appointment if you need one.

➤ Look favorably on a plan with high rates of preventive care delivery.

➤ Look closely at high or low rates of hospitalization and surgery. Compare them with some appropriate norm or standard. Very high rates could signal a plan authorizing unnecessary care or care that is made necessary by poor patient management. Very low rates may mean that the plan heavily rations its services.

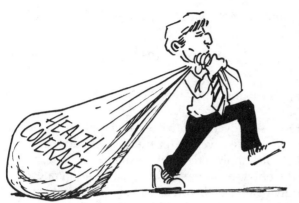

Chapter 7

Passages: From Job to Job, and from Job to the Unknown

In This Chapter

➤ Changing jobs? You can take your coverage with you.

➤ New beginnings: Keeping your coverage in a new job or when you strike out on your own

➤ It's all in the family, but let your plan know

Everybody knows that people without health care coverage can have problems getting the care they need. But people with coverage can have problems, too. Many are afraid to change jobs—or strike out in business on their own—because they or their family members could lose part or all of their coverage by moving to a new plan.

There are now laws that set up new ways to stretch the coverage that *is* offered by employers. But fair warning: No law requires an employer to offer health care coverage in the first place.

Whether you get your care from a managed care plan or a fee-for-service plan, this chapter gives you the information you need to sustain health care coverage when you are on your own, between jobs, or starting a new one. In this chapter, we focus on the broad outlines of these protections and the special issues they pose for managed care plan participants. If these changes happen to you, read and understand everything your plan sends you.

You Can Take It with You

Most firms that do offer health coverage must comply with two important laws that extend coverage beyond the work place:

➤ The Consolidated Omnibus Budget Reconciliation Act of 1985, commonly known as COBRA

➤ The Health Insurance Portability and Accountability Act of 1996, or HIPAA

COBRA requires employers with 20 or more employees to offer certain employees who are leaving their jobs the right to continue health care coverage for themselves and their dependents at their own expense. Parallel rules apply to employees of federal, state, and local governments. COBRA coverage is the only way to remain covered at group rates, which are much more favorable than individual rates. If you leave your job, the documents you receive from your health plan or your employer will probably use the term COBRA. Many states have COBRA–like regulations that apply to even smaller firms or have longer periods of coverage; your documents should mention these requirements as well, since you are entitled to whichever coverage is more generous.

HIPAA, on the other hand, established *portability* rules that help two more groups get and keep coverage:

➤ Those who have trouble buying or keeping health care coverage due to health problems

➤ Those whose plans do not cover health care conditions they or their dependents were treated for before joining the plan (pre-existing conditions)

Healthspeak
Federal *portability* rules make it easier for people to carry their health coverage from job to job and from group plans to individual coverage.

These laws require employers and sometimes insurance companies and health care plans to inform you of your rights to access and sustain health care coverage. Both the continued coverage and portability laws are complicated enough that we can't cover all the possible situations you could encounter in this chapter. But you need to know enough to protect yourself by having a general idea of your rights and important deadlines you and your plan must meet. If you don't, you may miss out on coverage you are supposed to be offered. Missed opportunities can cost you money, your health, and even your life.

We're going to follow a family—Bea Wilder, her husband, and kids—through some of the situations that arise under COBRA and HIPAA. The picture below depicts their progress through the system.

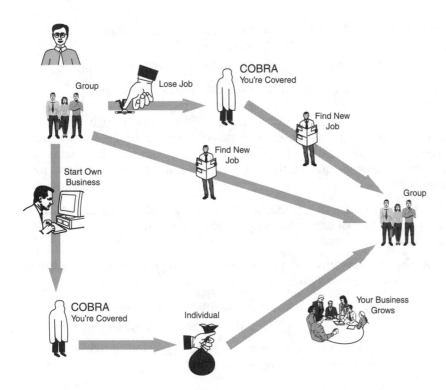

Your paths through the health care system.

When You Lose Your Job: What Next?

Both continued coverage and portability rules come into play when you leave your job, whether or not you go back to work again. The two laws work together. Be careful: Forgoing your rights under one law may make the other law's protections useless, or at least less useful.

Your Rights to Continued Coverage

If your employer is covered by COBRA (remember, some small firms are not) and you have health care coverage, you, your dependents, (including your spouse) or both have the right to continued coverage if:

➤ You leave your job, get laid off, retire, or are fired (other than for gross misconduct)

➤ Your hours are reduced, leading to a loss of coverage (strikers are included under this clause)

➤ You die

➤ You are divorced or legally separated from your spouse (simply agreeing to live apart does not count; more on divorce later in this chapter)

➤ You become entitled to Medicare (your spouse may be younger or you may have dependent children who qualify for COBRA coverage)

➤ Your child ceases to be a qualifying dependent under the terms of the plan

➤ A child is born to or adopted by you while you are on COBRA coverage

People who lose coverage for the first two reasons are entitled to buy coverage for 18 months from the date of the event that caused their loss of coverage; others are entitled to 36 months of coverage. For Bea and her husband, her reduction to part-time status caused her to become ineligible for the health plan, but they could still buy coverage for the next 18 months.

Children born while their parent(s) are COBRA beneficiaries themselves become beneficiaries for the length of the normal eligibility period. Before, the child would have lost those rights if the covered parent died.

There are special rules on the duration of coverage, under which you may get more time, and even lifetime, coverage. They apply to:

➤ Retirees who lose coverage as a result of the bankruptcy of their former employer

➤ People who are disabled at the time they become eligible for COBRA coverage

➤ People who experience more than one of the events listed previously (you lose your job, and then you and your spouse divorce, for example)

Caution
You lose COBRA eligibility if you stop making your premium payments, and your eligibility cannot be reinstated, even if you make up the arrears.

So, when Mrs. Bea Wilder's husband suffered a debilitating heart attack during his period of eligibility, the only up side was that special rules now applied to their coverage.

Now you are stuck with the benefits you chose during your last open enrollment period, instead of that fancy new plan your employer just set up. Right? Wrong. As a COBRA beneficiary, you have the same coverage rights as an active employee, including the right to change, add, or eliminate coverage during an open enrollment period your employer may offer.

Be prepared for sticker shock. Your employer may charge you up to 102 percent of the total cost of keeping you in the plan. If your employer pays all or most of the cost of your coverage as an active employee, COBRA coverage (anywhere from $3,000 to $5,000 per year for family coverage) could be a big bite out of your budget. And, while health care premiums paid by an employer are not taxable income to the covered employee, many people will not get any tax benefits for their COBRA payments. But if all your employer is currently doing is providing you access to coverage at group rates (no small thing given the cost of many individual plans), your coverage costs under COBRA may not rise by much.

When Your COBRA Bites the Dust

You lose your COBRA coverage once your period of eligibility ends. In the past, you could have been denied coverage when you then chose to buy individual or family coverage on your own. Under HIPAA, though, you are now guaranteed the right to buy—and renew—coverage on your own as long as you meet these conditions:

➤ You have had at least 18 months of almost any type of health care coverage, including Medicaid.

➤ Your most recent coverage was under a group plan.

➤ You have exhausted your COBRA rights or similar rights you may have under state law.

➤ You keep up your premiums.

You may be able to buy this coverage through the same insurer that covered you in your previous job and during your COBRA days, or you may be able to go to a new insurer. Depending on the state where you live, you may be able to enter a state program designed to guarantee individuals access to health care coverage rather than requiring insurance companies to guarantee that enrollees can buy and renew coverage. Some states—perhaps as many as 30—may choose to set up separate risk pools for this purpose. Your state's insurance commissioner will tell you whether this option is available in your state (check your phone book for the insurance commissioner's consumer hot line in your state).

What do you lose? You lose the 102 percent ceiling on cost and the advantage of group coverage. What do you gain? You gain access to coverage. Though it may be costly, if you or a family member has a preexisting condition that requires frequent or costly care, consider making the sacrifice to buy individual coverage rather than being uninsured. Once you become re-employed, the time you had individual coverage counts toward any preexisting condition limitations your new employer's plan may impose.

Following the Wilders here, Bea continued buying coverage after her COBRA benefits ended. Even though the premiums were high, she still had health care coverage for her family, including her sickly husband.

Your Personal Rx
The amount you have to pay for individual coverage is regulated by the states. Insurance companies selling individual coverage policies may continue to limit or exclude coverage for preexisting conditions only until January 1, 1998, in most states. But some states may have longer to comply with federal law. Check with your insurance agent or your state's Department of Insurance.

Caution
Most plans come under the HIPAA requirements by 1998, but a small portion do not have to comply until 1999 or 2000. If health care coverage is important to your decision to change jobs, you may want to ask a new employer some questions before signing on the dotted line.

A New Start: Follow the HIPAA Trail

Congratulations! You've landed on your feet, with a new job that offers health care coverage. Exit old plan, enter new plan. Your new employer's plan may limit or exclude coverage for preexisting conditions; it's still allowed. What has changed is whether or not these limitations or exclusions will affect *you*.

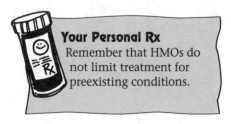

Your Personal Rx
Remember that HMOs do not limit treatment for preexisting conditions.

Under the new portability rules, limitations may generally not last longer than 12 months. People who have had no breaks in health care coverage—or a break lasting 62 days or less—receive a credit against such limitations of one month for each month of prior coverage. Such credits can be based on just about any coverage, including another employer plan, COBRA, individual coverage, or a government plan such as Medicaid.

If you have a preexisting condition, enroll in your employer's plan as soon as possible. Otherwise, the plan may be able to deny or limit coverage for preexisting conditions for up to 18 months. And until the plan becomes subject to the new portability rules, it may be able to deny you coverage entirely based on your health history.

When Bea Wilder accepted her new post at Wisdom Industries, she enrolled in her new employer's plan as soon as possible. In fact, she talked to the human resources department to make sure she was clear on when to sign up. Because she had continuous coverage from the time she was with her former employer and her COBRA coverage, coverage for her husband's heart condition was assured within a month.

New Options for the Self-Employed and Small Businesses

So you've decided to pursue the dream of wage slaves everywhere—you've signed on to be your own boss! The new portability rules require insurance companies to do special things that affect you, too:

➤ Insurers that offer coverage in the small group market must now offer to any small employers all the products they actively sell in a particular market.

➤ Insurers can require that the employer make at least a minimum contribution to the employees' premiums and that the plan achieve at least a minimum level of participation by eligible employees.

➤ Insurers marketing to the small group market must also accept all eligible individuals without regard to their health status.

These provisions may apply not only to owners of small businesses wanting to find health care coverage for their employees, but also to the mad genius starting the next Xerox or IBM in his garage. The new federal portability rules do not apply to plans that have fewer than two participants who are current employees (others could be family members). But some states consider plans with fewer than two employees to be group plans, so that your state's group insurance law provisions could give you similar protections to those available under federal law.

If you don't join another group health plan and aren't interested in—or can't afford—individual coverage, you may have other ways to find coverage.

You may be eligible for health care coverage because you are a member of a professional association, industry association, the Chamber of Commerce, or one of many other groups small employers and the self-employed may join. Under HIPAA, these plans will have to meet laws governing group coverage, including using prior coverage to offset preexisting condition limitations and banning discrimination among applicants based on health status.

If Your Employer Changes Plans

One thing is certain in health care: As soon as you learn the rules, they change. If the change amounts just to adding a new option, like adding a Point of Service plan to your HMO (see Chapter 1 for an explanation of this), you should generally be able to change to that option during your employer's open enrollment period, whether you are receiving benefits as an active employee or under COBRA.

But if the employer gets rid of your plan entirely in favor of a new plan, bad things can happen. The new plan's benefits may not be as generous as in your previous plan, and your out-of-pocket costs could increase substantially.

Just when Bea thought her health care problems were behind her, Wisdom Industries changed to PANES Health Care and increased her copay from $10 for a specialist visit to $40 per visit. Her out-of-pocket expenses the next month increased from $40 to $160.

If your employer gets rid of your health care plan and does not offer a new one, whether you are eligible for COBRA benefits depends on what happens to your employer:

➤ If the employer drops the plan completely but stays in business, COBRA benefits do not apply.

➤ A plant closing does not trigger COBRA eligibility either, unless the employer maintains other health plans, say for other plants or divisions.

➤ If the company is sold, the buyer, the seller, or both may be liable for offering COBRA benefits to any employees who lose their jobs in the transaction.

➤ If the company files bankruptcy, retirees and surviving spouses as of the date of bankruptcy are

Your Personal Rx

You do not usually become eligible for COBRA benefits if your employer changes or even terminates your health care plan. The employer has an obligation to give you notice of such changes (ask if you suspect changes; some slip up!), and you may have rights to continued benefits under state law.

entitled to lifetime COBRA coverage (more on this in Chapter 8). But if no health plan exists after the bankruptcy filing, employees who may lose their jobs have no COBRA rights.

If you lose coverage because your plan is terminated, your employer goes out of business, or both, you should find out whether you are eligible for *conversion coverage*, available directly from your insurance company or managed care plan, under your plan's provisions. If you are eligible, you would not need to show evidence of good health, but your conversion benefits may be fewer, your costs higher, or both, compared with your group coverage.

Healthspeak

Conversion coverage, which allows you to buy health care coverage after you are no longer eligible for group or COBRA coverage, is purchased directly from your insurance company or managed care plan.

What's Bea Wilder to do when her company goes through these changes? Keep on top of what's happening. Talk (and write) often to the human resources department, making a list of the information she has requested. Get her own information on how long she has been covered and on payroll deductions for health insurance. She may need it to assert her rights to coverage. These can be difficult times.

Family Matters

Your health care coverage needs to change as your family changes. Here are some things to consider as your family grows or shrinks.

Wedding Bells and Stork Visits

If you get married, give birth, or adopt a child, or if your spouse loses his or her own coverage, you have a right to ask your plan to cover your spouse or child. Some plans already let you do this, without making you wait for an open enrollment period, as long as you give them prompt notice (usually 30 days from the event). Prompt notice usually exempts the person you add from preexisting condition limitations or the requirement to provide evidence of good health.

The federal portability rules we discussed earlier will require most plans to allow new spouses or children to enroll promptly. Unless the plan provides otherwise, the new enrollee can be required to serve the preexisting condition limitation period, though prior coverage can be used to offset it. These new enrollees, however, unlike those who decided not to enroll for other reasons, are subject to a maximum limitation period of 12, not 18, months.

D-I-V-O-R-C-E

If you're divorced, you probably know first hand that your health care and other employee benefits should be explicitly dealt with in a divorce agreement. Let's move on to the logistics of getting care for children when you and your ex-spouse share custody, whether routinely or for extended visits. Divorce is not easy; making mistakes with your health care coverage makes it that much harder.

You can usually cover a stepchild in your employer's plan, even if you have not legally adopted the child. The child has to live with you in a parent-child relationship, and you have to support the child. Some plans require that you or your current spouse be able to claim the child as a dependent for tax purposes.

But even the most amicable joint-custody arrangement can fail to take account of the intricacies of managed care plans. Suppose you are the stepmother, and the child is covered under your policy. Will you share all the plan information with your stepchild's mother? Will your husband do it? If an emergency arises while the child is visiting her mother, will you seek the plan's approval for needed care? Will your stepchild's mother do it? Will your husband do it?

Agree on all this ahead of time. Otherwise, the parent or stepparent without the plan information at hand may make mistakes that risk not only large sums of money, but also the child's health and even life.

Divorce can complicate COBRA benefits if you are in an HMO or similar plan. If Bea Wilder divorces her husband and he and their children move outside the plan's service area, the HMO is not useful to them, but their COBRA coverage may still be. If Wisdom Industries has other employees in their new community, the spouse and children have to be offered the same coverage as employees in that area. But if her employer has no employees in that area, the spouse and children have two options:

➤ The right to choose other coverage (if such coverage is available to active employees) when open enrollment season comes around

➤ The right to buy individual coverage on the open market without exhausting their period of COBRA eligibility

> **Your Personal Rx**
> If you are in an HMO or similar program, no longer live or work in its service area, and have no other COBRA alternatives available to you, your COBRA coverage is considered exhausted even if the full amount of time you could have bought it has not elapsed. This allows you to buy guaranteed coverage in the individual market.

What Is a Dependent Child?

Back in the dark ages (when we were in college, that is), most people started college at 18 or so, stayed for four years, graduated, and bought cars. Today, kids still buy cars, but everything else has changed. Many wait for a few years after high school before deciding whether college is for them. Others enroll right after high school, but may take five to six years to finish a degree. Many are enrolled only as part-time students.

Parents of long-term scholars need to know what their health plan provisions are with respect to dependent children (see Chapter 20). First, plans typically require that your children be unmarried to be covered under your plan. Second, the child must generally be under 19 years of age. The age limit may be extended to 23 if the child is enrolled in school and depends solely on you for support. A disabled, dependent child may be eligible for coverage even if older than these limits if the disability occurred while the child was still eligible as a dependent. Because your child's coverage depends on the precise wording of your plan, read the plan contract to evaluate gaps in his or her coverage.

Caution

Once your child is married or is older than the plan limit for dependent coverage, his or her coverage under your plan is generally terminated. You or your child should explore COBRA coverage if no other coverage is available.

Not that your plan doesn't trust you, but it almost always needs official confirmation of your student's status. Once your student is enrolled in school, ask the school's registrar to send a Proof of Enrollment letter to your plan (and a copy to you). You may have to do this each year. Check your member handbook or with member services to find out where and to whom to send the letter. Check later to make sure your plan has the letter on record.

Your Rights

From the first day you are covered under an employer-sponsored health care coverage plan, you have a right to:

➤ Information about your plan

➤ Notice if your right to be covered changes

➤ Time to make certain decisions if your life circumstances change

➤ More time

Your rights to continued coverage and portability of your benefits are enforced by severe monetary penalties on employers. But your rights may depend on whether you have fulfilled your obligations.

Information

Employers get substantial tax benefits from sponsoring health plans. In exchange, the federal government requires them to give you enough information to know how to use your plan and make sure it is operated correctly (more on this in Chapter 3). This obligation does not end when you are no longer an employee. COBRA beneficiaries are entitled to all the information available to employees, including notice of changes in benefits and premiums, open enrollment seasons, and annual reports. You and your covered dependents are required to be informed of your COBRA rights upon first enrolling in the employer's plan.

Make sure you get the COBRA information. Keep an eye on your COBRA rights, whether you plan to stay one year or 20. You never know when you might need it.

Remember reading about how you can offset the time you must wait to cover a preexisting condition with the time you were covered under your old plan? There are a few steps to make this work, and the onus is not always on you:

➤ Once the portability rules apply to your plan, it must notify you if it has preexisting condition terms and offer to help you get proof of prior coverage.

➤ Your previous plan and the insurer or organization that provided coverage are also obligated to provide you and your dependents with proof of your prior coverage. They have to coordinate who provides proof, not you.

➤ Your new plan must also notify you if your coverage history is not long enough to completely exempt you from the preexisting condition limitations and give you the chance to submit more evidence.

Notice

Unlike most of the other rights in this section, the right to notice goes both ways between you and your employer. Your employer will know when you've quit, died, been fired, or had your hours reduced. You have the right to receive written notice of your right to elect COBRA coverage when one of these events occurs.

You have the obligation to inform the employer of other events in your life, such as a divorce, that would make you or a family member eligible for continued (COBRA) coverage or for regular coverage under your plan or your spouse's plan under the portability rules.

Time

The laws governing your health benefit rights recognize that the decisions you face are sometimes complicated and require time to make. After all, these decisions accompany difficult events, such as job loss, marriage or divorce, and death, all of which are demanding on their own. Here are some important deadlines you need to know:

➤ You usually have a month from the date you become eligible for your employer's plan to pick a plan. After that time, you may be required to present evidence of good health to be covered (until your plan is subject to the portability rules).

➤ You usually have a month to cover a new spouse or child under your plan. Plans that don't permit this now will have to do so once the portability rules kick in.

➤ You must notify your employer of a divorce or other event that would make you or a dependent eligible for COBRA coverage within 60 days of the event itself or the date when your coverage would end, whichever is later.

➤ You or your eligible dependents usually have 60 days to decide whether to accept COBRA coverage.

➤ Once you have made a COBRA decision (called an *election*), you have 45 days to make your first premium payment for the period between the event that led to your eligibility and the date you made your election.

➤ After your COBRA coverage expires, you usually have a month to decide whether to accept conversion (basically, individual) coverage under the plan.

So, when you receive the plan paperwork from your new employer or notification of your COBRA rights, you don't have to fill them out right away, but don't delay too long, and keep an eye on the calendar.

More Time

In general, the deadlines listed in the previous section are firm. But sometimes you get a break. For continued coverage, for example, you have a grace period of 30 days to make your premium from the date the premium is otherwise due.

Watch the Paperwork and the Calendar

We can't emphasize this enough: Watch the paperwork! Make sure of your rights as outlined in this chapter and get the information you need to claim them.

Watch the calendar. Most deadlines for obtaining or preserving your health care coverage are *not* extendable. As soon as you learn of a deadline, put it on your calendar a week or two before the deadline to ensure you make it. If you send payments or other documents or information, use overnight or registered mail so that you have a receipt. If you slip up, you bear the consequences.

The Least You Need to Know

➤ If you have health care coverage, your employer must let you and your dependents stay in the plan for a period of time after your hours are reduced, you stop working entirely, you die, become eligible for Medicare, or certain changes in your family status occur. Employers with fewer than 20 employees are exempt from this require-ment.

➤ Once your COBRA coverage is exhausted, insurers, including HMOs, are required to sell you an individual policy (or one for your family) if you want one.

➤ If you move to a new group plan or to individual coverage, your prior coverage—including continued coverage under COBRA—can count against preexisting condi-tion limitations in the new plan if you have not had substantial breaks in coverage.

➤ Marriage, divorce, a new child, or the independence of a grown child can mean changes in your coverage needs and rights.

➤ If your employer terminates your health care plan, goes out of business, or both, you may have rights to continued health care coverage under state law.

➤ Watch the health care coverage deadlines when your family status changes. Miss a deadline, and your rights are lost.

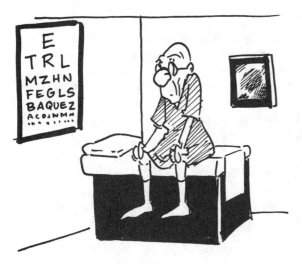

Chapter 8

Managed Care
for Seniors

In This Chapter

➤ Coverage options after 65

➤ Is a managed care plan the right choice for you?

➤ Finding out if your coverage travels with you

➤ What to think about when you make your choice

➤ Finding help when you need it

It's Tuesday afternoon, and you're busy being retired. After golf, you head over to the Historical Society where you help set up for the evening program. Next week you'll work 10 hours at the bookstore and start a history course at the local college. Friday finds you on the plane for a three-day weekend in Orlando. Health care lurks in the back of your mind, but you have Medicare.

Nearly all people age 65 or older—and some younger—are covered under Medicare, the health care component of the Social Security program. But this does not mean that health care choices get simpler for retirees. While Medicare is a good program, it does not cover all the medical care the typical retiree will need. In particular, outpatient prescription drugs (drugs for in-hospital use are covered as part of hospital care coverage) is an important component of spending for the elderly, and one often not covered by any kind of insurance. Medicare also requires copayments and deductibles for covered care, which can add up over time.

Your Personal Rx

The federal government publishes *Your Medicare Handbook*, available at no charge (Medicare enrollees receive this automatically). This book is a user-friendly explanation of who is eligible for Medicare, how to enroll, what expenses are covered, and the major features of Medigap and managed care plans. Use it as a starting point in figuring out your needs.

Your Personal Rx

Most people do not qualify for Medicare until age 65, even if they have retired from their principal job or have a spouse who is 65. If your employer offers you early retirement, find out if you get health care coverage until you reach Medicare eligibility, and what, if anything, you will get as a Medicare supplement.

To fill in these gaps, retirees generally get health care coverage from one or more additional sources: their former employer, the private insurance market (these plans are called Medigap plans, because they fill in Medicare's gaps), or Medicaid, the joint federal-state health care coverage program for low-income persons. Both Medicare and many of these additional coverage sources may require retirees to choose their health plan.

This chapter will tell you how managed care can figure in your health care planning after age 65. It won't tell you everything you need to know about Medicare—there are other publications for that—but it will walk you through the major health care coverage choices you will face in retirement.

Your Health Care Coverage Options

As a group, the 65+ population spends more on health care—and more out of their own pockets—than any other age group. For example, the average retiree can expect to spend nearly $50 per month, and more than one in ten will spend over $100 per month.

Medicare

Medicare has two parts. Part A covers hospital care, and Part B covers physician care and other outpatient services. Everyone who reaches age 65 and has accumulated the necessary number of years of covered employment (currently 40 quarters or 10 years) is eligible to participate in both. Dependent widows or widowers of covered employees may begin participating in Medicare at age 62. Part A is free; Part B requires a monthly premium that changes yearly. This premium is $43.80 per month per person for 1997.

Not everyone pays Medicare payroll taxes in their principal job. Many state and local government workers are a prominent example. If you don't have enough covered quarters under Medicare, you don't get coverage. But many people who do not pay Medicare taxes in their main job do so in a second job or have spouses who do so, and get coverage that way.

Medicaid

Medicaid is the joint federal-state program providing health care coverage for low-income persons (see Chapter 10). Two groups of Medicare beneficiaries with low incomes and few assets may qualify for Medicaid assistance in paying their health care costs:

➤ The Qualified Medicare Beneficiary (QMB) program pays Medicare premiums, deductibles, and coinsurance for certain elderly and disabled persons who are entitled to Medicare Part A. Your income must be at or below the national poverty level (this level varies by the size of the household and is updated annually), and your savings and assets cannot exceed $4,000 for one person or $6,000 for a couple.

➤ If your income is too high to qualify for the QMB program, you may still qualify for the Specified Low-Income Medicare Beneficiary (SLMB) program. This program pays the Medicare Part B premium for people meeting the income requirements. Your state or local Medicaid, public welfare, or social services can give you more information and help you determine whether you qualify.

Employer Coverage

The roles of Medicare and employer-provided health care coverage in paying your bills differ according to whether you continue to work after age 65.

If You're Working

Many people who continue to work after age 65 don't see any reason to apply for Medicare. But if your employer does not offer health care coverage to active employees, or offers coverage that requires significant out-of-pocket outlays such as deductibles or copayments, there is no reason not to sign up at least for Part A of Medicare when you turn 65.

But take note: Your Part B premiums go up by ten percent for every year that you could have been enrolled but were not. As a result, people who delay retirement may be especially interested in enrolling in a Medicare HMO.

If you are covered by your employer's health care plan, you may not need to enroll in Part B while you are working. The employer plan remains *primary payor* for employed Medicare beneficiaries, as well as for participants who are disabled and have health care coverage through their employer or that of a family

Your Personal Rx
The Health Care Financing Administration (HCFA), the federal agency that administers Medicare and Medicaid, advises that you apply for Part A of Medicare three months before you turn 65.

Healthspeak
The primary payor pays its share of covered expenses first, while the secondary payor pays some or all of the amounts left over. So if your employer plan is primary it will typically pay $80 of a $100 doctor bill, and Medicare will pay $20. But employer plans interact with Medicare in various ways, and your out-of-pocket costs could be higher than in this example.

Caution
Hospitals, doctors, and other health care providers—social workers, nutritionists, and others—must submit Medicare claims for you. To save money, make sure they know about all other benefits for which you may be eligible.

member, or are entitled to workers' compensation, federal black lung benefits, no-fault insurance, or liability insurance. Special rules also apply to kidney dialysis patients covered by an employer group health plan and to people eligible for both Medicare and veterans benefits. Which plan is primary for you will affect the paperwork you have to do to be reimbursed for your health care expenses.

If You're Retired

Many people whose employer offers health care coverage to active employees are able to stay with that plan when they retire. They may have to pay a premium to do so. The coverage is typically identical to that offered active employees. There is one major difference: Medicare is the primary payor for Medicare enrollees who are no longer covered as active employees.

If you are in a PPO, IPA, or certain other plans, Medicare "sees" you as a fee-for-service plan enrollee. So, if you plan to stay in the plan's service area, you probably don't need to do anything other than inform the plan that you are participating in Medicare. Your provider will bill Medicare directly, with your plan paying some of the charges that Medicare does not cover and you paying the rest.

If you are not already in a managed care plan, your employer may encourage you to enroll in one when you retire.

COBRA Coverage for Retirees

Medicare is a good health care plan but leaves some important gaps, notably prescription drug coverage. Therefore, if your employer does not continue your coverage after you retire, you may want to continue to participate in your employer's plan after retirement. COBRA (Consolidated Omnibus Reconciliation Act; see Chapter 7) coverage may be especially of interest to you if you retire before you are eligible for Medicare. You may be eligible to do so:

➤ If your employer's retiree health benefit ends when you become eligible for Medicare at age 65, you may generally elect COBRA coverage under your former employer's plan for up to three years.

➤ If you are disabled at the time you become eligible for COBRA coverage, you may purchase coverage for 29 months. This ensures you coverage until your Medicare benefits begin (at a cost of up to 150 percent of the applicable premium after the initial 18 months).

➤ If you become eligible for COBRA coverage because your company goes bankrupt *and* you are retired at the time the bankruptcy occurs, you and your spouse are eligible to purchase coverage for life.

COBRA coverage is at your expense unless the plan provides otherwise and may cost up to 102 percent of what it costs the employer to include you in the plan (for more on COBRA, see Chapter 7).

Be careful about electing COBRA coverage if you have a chronic health condition, such as diabetes, high blood pressure, or heart trouble. Such a medical condition could make it difficult for you to obtain Medigap coverage to supplement Medicare after your COBRA coverage expires, since insurers can check up on your health after you have been on Medicare for six months.

If you have a chronic condition that could make it difficult for you to get coverage and wait to look for it until your COBRA eligibility period runs out, a Medicare HMO may be your best bet. HMOs with Medicare contracts may not conduct medical pre-screening, making them potentially good choices for people with chronic health problems (but see "Even More Things to Think About," later in this chapter).

Medigap

Many people choose to buy private insurance, called Medigap, to supplement Medicare. The federal government requires that Medigap policies follow one of ten standardized models, lettered A through J, shown in the table on the following page. All insurers offering Medigap policies are required to offer plan A (the basic package) and may offer the others at their discretion. Each individual plan must be the same, regardless of the insurer selling it.

The various plans differ significantly in their coverage for such items as stays in a skilled nursing facility, emergency medical care overseas, prescription drugs, and other items. Their annual costs to you will differ significantly as well. The price for each package may also vary from insurer to insurer. For example, in 1997, depending on where you live, your age, and the plan you select, you could be paying as little as $300 per year for a basic A plan or as much as $3,000 per year for the J plan. Evaluate each policy carefully.

Healthspeak

Under *entry-age rating*, your premium is higher the older you are upon entering the plan but does not change as you age. Under *attained-age rating*, your premium increases every year. Attained-age rating can make a big difference in your budget if your employer pension is not indexed for inflation (most government pensions are, but most private pensions are not).

An HMO is not allowed to vary premiums based on the age of the enrollee. In contrast, Medigap plans in most states may use *entry-age rating* (your premium depends on your age when you enter the plan) or *attained-age rating* (your premium depends on your current age). As this book was written, ten states prohibited attained-age rating. If you are interested in Medigap coverage (rather than a Medicare HMO), check with your local Medicare office to see what the law is in your state.

Key Features of Medigap Plans

Benefit	Plan [1]									
	A	B	C	D	E	F	G	H	I	J
Core Benefits [2]	X	X	X	X	X	X	X	X	X	X
SNF Coinsurance	—	—	X	X	X	X	X	X	X	X
Part A Deductible	—	X	X	X	X	X	X	X	X	X
Part B Deductible	—	—	X	—	—	X	—	—	—	X
Part B Excess charges [3]	—	—	—	—	H	L	—	—	H	H
Foreign travel	—	—	X	X	X	X	X	X	X	X
At home recovery	—	—	—	X	—	—	X	—	X	X
Prescription drugs [4]	—	—	—	—	—	—	—	L	L	H
Preventive care	—	—	—	—	X	—	—	—	—	X
% of sales [5]	5.1	17.1	21.2	8.4	0.8	29.7	2.2	2.7	5.9	6.9

Source: McCormack et al. (1996).

1/: Plans are the 10 uniform benefit packages mandated under federal law. "X" means the benefit is offered;—means it is not.

2/: Include coverage of all Part A (hospital) coinsurance for stays longer than 60 days, part B coinsurance, Parts A and B blood deductible, and the 365 lifetime reserve days of hospital care.

3/: Low coverage pays 80 percent and high coverage pays 100 percent of the difference between the physician's charge and the Medicare-allowable rate.

4/: Low coverage has a $250 annual deductible, 50 percent coinsurance, and a maximum annual benefit of $1,250; high coverage has the same deductible and coinsurance but a $3,000 maximum annual benefit.

5/: In Florida, Missouri, New York, South Carolina, Texas, and Washington.

Remember, too, that you are making a decision for the long term. At age 65, foreign travel coverage could be more important to you than prescription drug coverage if you are in good health. In 5 or 10 years, however, you may face different needs. Based on insurance data collected in six states, plans B, C, and F together account for more than half of all Medigap policy sales.

Is a Managed Care Plan Right for You?

Whether you should consider managed care depends in part on your own attitudes and personality. Most people find that their choice of doctors and treatments is more limited in managed care plans than in traditional fee-for-service plans. Such limits could be more important to seniors, because many of us accumulate both health conditions and long histories with our doctors by the time we reach a certain age.

House Call

Managed care patients need to be their own advocates. Managed care is another large organization for seniors to deal with, just when they are dealing with Social Security and Medicare—other large systems. Older patients are often not used to being in charge of their health care and are used to a system of unlimited choice. The trade-off, once again, is less choice for more savings.

On the other hand, most people now planning for retirement will have had at least some experience with managed care, utilization review, or both prior to retirement. Those who recently retired may be better able to function in a managed care environment than those who are much older and experienced only with fee-for-service plans.

Whether you can sign up in a Medicare HMO depends on where you live. As this book was written, about three in four Medicare beneficiaries lived in areas served by at least one Medicare HMO, and more than half had a choice of at least two plans, but nine states had no Medicare HMOs. Enrollment remains highly concentrated, with California, Florida, and Arizona accounting for 60 percent of Medicare HMO enrollment (but only 19 percent of all Medicare beneficiaries).

Your regional HCFA office may have a comparison chart showing the benefits available and the premiums charged by the Medicare HMOs offered in its region. The following table summarizes the main features of benefits available in 42 Medicare HMOs in Arizona, California, Nevada, and southeastern Pennsylvania, and compares these benefits with those available under traditional Medicare. For details and up-to-date information about the plans in your area, contact your regional HCFA offices or the managed care plans of interest to you.

A Comparison of Traditional Medicare and Medicare HMO Benefits in a Sample of 42 Medicare HMOs

Feature	Medicare	Medicare HMOs Feature	#	Remarks
Premiums/month	Part B = $42.50	$0	40	Includes HMOs that charged premiums in addition to Part B only in some service areas.
Hospital	Varies by days used, up to 150 days	Full, unlimited days	42	2 HMOs required a copayment for use of unaffiliated hospitals and required 4 emergencies or referrals.
Physicians/ Specialists	20%, $100 deductible/year	$0–$10 per visit	42	
Skilled Nursing Facility	After 3 days in hospital, first 20 days no charge, 21–100 days $92/day	At least 100 days	42	8 required prior hospitalizations or referrals.
Home Health Care	No charge	No charge	42	1 offered respite care.
Emergency room				Plans that do not
In area	20%, $100 deductible	$0 or waived w/admit	36	waive ER charges either impose a flat
Out of area	20%, $100 deductible	$0 or waived w/admit	36	fee or cover them under hospital
Worldwide	Not covered	$0 or waived w/admit	36	coverage.
Preventive Care	Not covered			
Exam		$0–$10	42	6 plans only every 2 years.
Eye glasses		Covered	39	Discount, co-payment, or allowance.
Routine vision exam		Covered	40	24 plans only every 2 years.
Routine hearing exam		Covered	37	
Hearing aids		Covered	19	Discount or allowance.
Pharmacy	Not covered	Covered	41	Generally copayment of $3–$10 with an annual cap on benefits.

Feature	Medicare	Medicare HMOs Feature	#	Remarks
Routine Dental	Not covered	Coverage offered	30	
Mental health	See hospital coverage			
Inpatient	190 lifetime days	No charge	36	
Outpatient	50%, $100 deductible	190 life-time days	36 42	

Source: Authors' calculations based on data provided by HCFA.

A word of caution: Managed care plans are in fierce competition for you and your Medicare dollars. You are among the fastest growing group of HMO enroll- ees. You may benefit if you have more than one HMO in your area. The areas included in our summary had more than two HMOs, so benefits in these areas may be more generous than in areas with little competi- tion among managed care plans. Use the table above as a guide, not the last word, to the benefits you should expect:

Your Personal Rx
A national HMO comparison chart will be made available on the HCFA Website (check the tearout card at the front of this book) as well as by mail in late 1997 or early 1998.

➤ Most of the HMOs we surveyed did not charge premiums in addition to Medicare Part B, and all provided physician, hospital, and skilled nursing facility benefits.

➤ Most did not charge separately for emergency room services if the patient was admitted to the hospital, but those that did typically charged $50 or less.

➤ Preventive care and pharmacy benefits were widely available.

➤ Almost half of the HMOs provided assistance with hearing aid purchases.

➤ Routine dental coverage was offered by nearly three in four plans but was not included in their basic package, meaning you would typically have to pay more for it.

➤ Inpatient mental health care typically had the same limits as under traditional Medicare, but outpatient care was typically available for fixed fees ranging from $0 to $30 per visit.

Use both tables in this chapter to come up with your own action plan. There are trade- offs. In general, your out-of-pocket costs will be higher in most Medigap plans than in a Medicare HMO because most Medigap plans do not cover prescription drugs. You will also pay premiums in a Medigap plan and will generally face more paperwork. You have to balance costs, coverage, and paperwork against the restrictions on provider choice and possibly on treatments that you will face in a Medicare HMO.

Market conditions are changing rapidly, with HMOs entering new communities all the time. When you get ready to enroll in Medicare, check with your local Medicare office to see what is available to you.

Whether an HMO is what you need also depends in part on which coverage or combination of coverages you have.

If You Have Medicare (and Nothing Else)

There is no risk to you in trying an HMO, and you may get more benefits, lower your out-of-pocket costs, and reduce or eliminate health-related paperwork. By law, the Medicare HMO must cover Medicare *deductibles* and *copayments*, and it cannot reject you because of poor health or refuse to treat you for pre-existing conditions. If you decide you don't like the HMO, you can drop it and return to fee-for-service coverage on a monthly basis.

If You Have Medicare and Medigap

Your Personal Rx

If you want to try an HMO, particularly one that charges you no premiums, maintain your Medigap coverage until you are sure you like the HMO (after all, the HMO is not costing you anything). But cancel the Medigap policy if you decide to stay; you won't need a Medigap policy and won't be able to collect from it for care outside the HMO.

You need to be really sure that an HMO is what you want. Once you leave a Medigap plan, the plan has no obligation to take you back and, depending on your health history, might choose not to do so. Even if your medical chart is squeaky-clean and you have the blood pressure of an 18 year old, you have to consider the possibility that things could change.

If You Have Medicare and Employer Coverage

You can expect your employer to actively promote HMO enrollment. The reason is purely financial. If its Medicare-eligible retirees enroll in a "zero-premium" Medicare HMO contract—one that requires no payments from the employer or beneficiary—the employer's obligation is wiped out. HMOs can enroll Medicare participants "for free" because the Medicare program pays the HMO 95 percent of what it would cost the program to pay for traditional fee-for-service care in the HMO's service area.

To sweeten the deal for retirees, many employers will add to the basic benefits offered by the HMO. Such coverage will generally include such big-ticket items as outpatient prescription drug coverage; vision, dental, and hearing care; no deductibles; nominal copayments (or none at all); and no claims forms.

If you choose an HMO endorsed by your employer instead of fee-for-service coverage, make sure the benefits offered in the package are what you want and need, as your employer is deriving considerable financial benefit from enrolling you in it. Make sure that your employer formally acknowledges (in writing) your right to re-enter the fee-for-service plan if you change your mind.

If You Have Medicare and Medicaid

Look into enrolling in a Medicare HMO. Qualified Medical Beneficiaries (people eligible for Medicaid help with their Medicare payments) could receive better benefits—such as prescription drug benefits—while avoiding the need to file applications and send in forms and documents to show they are still eligible. Specified Low-Income Medicare Beneficiaries (other people eligible for Medicaid help with their Medicare payments) could eliminate paperwork, improve their benefits, and save money if they find a good zero-premium plan or one with premiums lower than the deductibles and coinsurance they must currently pay.

Double Trouble: Beware of Duplication

Health care coverage from more than one source can help you get the health care you need at a price you can afford. But you may be wasting your money because you won't always get benefits from lots of sources. If you have Medicare and a single Medigap policy, don't buy cancer insurance, hospital indemnity policies, or similar insurance, unless you know the additional insurance fills gaps in your coverage.

Caution
Long-term care insurance, which generally covers extended stays in a nursing home or similar facility, does not duplicate Medicare or Medigap coverage.

Snowbirds: Will Your Coverage Travel with You?

Now that you're retired, do you bypass the seasons you dislike by changing locale? If you enroll in a managed care plan, ask if you are covered during this period. The answer will depend on the type of plan you have and the length of time you plan to stay away from the plan's service area.

Medicare managed care requires you to learn a few terms that do not apply to other types of managed care. One type of Medicare HMO is called a risk plan. In a risk plan, as in any other type of HMO, you are locked into using the plan's providers unless the plan makes a referral elsewhere. Only urgent or emergency care is excepted from this rule. *Neither the plan nor Medicare* will generally pay for care you get outside the plan unless the situation is urgent or an emergency (for more on emergency and urgent care, see Chapter 14). In addition, if you spend 90 days or more outside the plan's service area, it can terminate your enrollment and leave you without coverage.

Your Personal Rx

If you are considering an HMO, ask about travel provisions. You may be able to obtain routine care at another facility. You might then have two or more doctors for the same condition. Make sure they know about each other and talk to each other when necessary.

Some risk plans offer *point-of-service* (POS) options that will cover a share of the cost of services obtained outside the plan. In return for this flexibility, you will have to pay at least 20 percent of the cost of the care.

Not all plans are the same. The federal government does not regulate the circumstances under which HMOs allow their members to go to non-network providers or the cost-sharing when outside providers are used. Look at the details of POS options when comparing plans and ask questions of the member services department.

Another type of HMO—less prevalent than risk plans—is the cost plan. Participants in this type of plan may use either affiliated (those that are part of the plan) or unaffiliated providers. The plan may not pay for care obtained from unaffiliated providers, but Medicare will.

Retirees and their families should also consider what will happen to their health care coverage if they move after retirement. Medicare, of course, is a national program, so benefits are available anywhere in the U.S. Make sure to file a change-of-address notification with your Medicare office when you move, so your claims get processed in the region where you live. HMO participants, however, will have to disenroll from their plan and either return to fee-for-service medicine or select a Medicare HMO in their new location if one is available.

Even More Things to Think About

Everyone—working or retired—needs to think cost, quality, location, and plan structure when making decisions about health care. Retirees need to add a few extras to that list.

Specialists

By the time you reach your retirement years, chances are you've had a few encounters with the health care system. If you select a managed care plan, pay particular attention to the availability and credentials of the specialists you need. Check to see if the plan has any specialists in geriatric medicine. Just as adults have different medical needs from those of children, so do adults' medical needs change as they age.

Location

Everyone should consider the location of a plan's facilities or providers in selecting a plan, but retirees should be especially careful. It may not be pleasant to think about the time when you may have to give up driving—and, indeed, you may never need to do so. But even the healthiest retirees or their spouses may be unable to drive during or after an ill-ness, injury, or surgery. Would you be able to reach your providers by public transportation, taxi, or rides from friends? Your health and speedy recovery could depend on your ability to get to follow-up appointments other than in your own car.

Plan Quality

Retirees should pay special attention to any measures of plan quality that show how well they treat chronic problems such as diabetes or hypertension. Ask questions about their plan's ability to help maintain their health with preventive care, such as whether they have geriatric specialists, or if some of their primary care doctors are trained in geriatric medicine (see Chapter 6 for a discussion of plan quality measures that can help you make this judgment).

Emergency Care

Everyone, but especially seniors, should know what their plan considers an emergency (more on this in Chapter 14). Some HMOs charge you a nominal fee if an emergency room visit does not result in a hospital admission; otherwise, the fee is waived.

Prescription Drug Limits

If you are in a health care plan that limits your prescription drug benefits, find out how the limit is formulated. It could be based on the retail price of the prescriptions you are using, on the pharmacy or other supplier's wholesale cost, or some other basis. Retail price is the least advantageous to you; other approaches may be better.

Help Is Available

When you sign up for Social Security and Medicare, you will receive easy-to-understand information explaining your benefits and rights. You can also call a toll-free number in your locality (check in the U.S. government pages of the phone book under "Medicare") with questions.

If you encounter a coverage, billing, or claim problem that you or the Medicare office can't solve, call your state insurance counseling and assistance (ICA) program. ICAs are available in all 50 states, the District of Columbia, and U.S. territories. There is no charge for this service (see your phone book or call your local Medicare office for the toll-free ICA number for your area).

> **Your Personal Rx**
> Your state counseling office can give you a free copy of the *Guide to Health Insurance for People with Medicare*. Use it as a starting point in figuring out what supplemental coverage you may need in retirement and what you should expect to pay for it.

The Least You Need to Know

➤ Explore your Medicare options before your 65th birthday, even if you plan on continuing to work, and *especially* if you do not have health care coverage through your employer.

➤ If you want supplemental (Medigap) coverage, buy your policy within six months of qualifying for Medicare. After this deadline, insurers can ask about your health before considering your application.

➤ If you leave a Medigap plan, you may not be able to reinstate your policy or get another one at a comparable price.

➤ If you have any health problems that cause you to be rejected for Medigap coverage, look into Medicare HMOs.

➤ If you spend more than 90 days a year out of your HMO's service area, you may lose your HMO coverage (you cannot lose your Medicare coverage).

➤ If you encounter problems in obtaining the care or the coverage you need, use the federally funded assistance available in your state.

Chapter 9

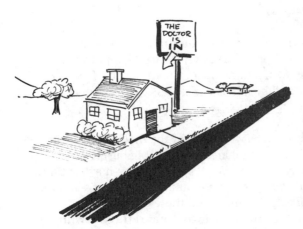

Beyond the Big City: Managed Care in Rural Areas

What does a farmer in northern Iowa have in common with a skipper on Cape Cod? Managed care.

Managed care is moving to *rural areas*, where about one in five Americans live, but it often looks different and works differently here from what is offered to urban residents. If you live in a rural area—and even if you only visit—this chapter will tell you what managed care means to you.

Many people think of rural life as healthy and safe, especially compared with the "mean streets" of many large American cities. This vision may be outdated. Rural residents are, indeed, less likely to die of homicide than city residents. However, rural residents are generally less healthy than urban residents and more likely to be injured, especially on the job. Higher injury rates reflect higher rates of employment in dangerous occupations, such as farming and mining, as well as higher rates of motor vehicle accidents due to longer travel distances. Rural incomes also tend to be lower than in urban areas, leading to lower rates of health care coverage and fewer health care providers.

Coming to an Area Near You

Managed care is on the move, so there is no place in the country that hasn't heard about it. Cost control, fueled by employers tired of price increases, led to the rapid spread of managed care. But health care costs in rural areas are low in the first place. Doctors and other health care professionals earn less, and hospitals charge less.

So who needs managed care beyond the big city?

Healthspeak

Rural areas are towns with fewer than 2,500 people, areas of open country, or counties with a central city (or twin cities) with fewer than 50,000 people. Areas on the outskirts of large cities are generally not considered rural.

Big business, that's who. One of the major forces bringing managed care to rural areas is those big businesses who have already tried various types of plans—maybe at headquarters, maybe at a city manufacturing plant—and found that it works for them. When these firms set up sites in rural areas, they bring their corporate attitudes with them. Once these big companies set up managed health plans for their employees in rural areas, it opens the way for others to join, too.

But the plans themselves aren't passive players in the move outside the city limits. Plans grow and are successful only by expanding their enrollment—their customer base. In large metropolitan areas, everybody is competing for numbers. Attracting members away from other plans requires advertising, promotions, price cuts, and benefit improvements, all of which cost money. A plan entering a rural area, on the other hand, may have the market all to itself (though entering a new market will cost it money, too).

The move into rural areas also makes it possible for plans to link urban markets. There can be as few as 20 miles or as many as 100 miles between cities large or small. Linking markets by expanding into the rural areas between them increases both a plan's potential membership and the resources available to its members.

And this can happen fast. An insurance agent from rural Virginia told us that watching managed care was like seeing a truck on the horizon. It seemed so far away but picked up speed so quickly that it nearly knocked her off the road when it whizzed past.

All well and good, but what does that mean to you? It means that the plan coming into *your* community and asking for *your* money, *your* trust, and power over *your* health may be driven there by factors having little or nothing to do with *you* and *your* needs. To even the playing field, you need to ask a few more questions about how the plan intends to serve you.

Rural Health Care Professionals

Doctors are the cornerstone of the health care system. This is true in urban and rural areas alike. But that is where the similarity ends. Rural doctors and other health care professionals are different from their urban brethren.

Rural Doctors

Some of the ways urban and rural doctors differ are measurable:

➤ Doctors are scarcer in rural areas than in urban areas.

➤ Rural doctors tend to be older. Many began their professional careers before *board certification* was widespread and would not meet the requirement of many managed care plans that doctors be board-certified or board-eligible.

➤ Rural doctors work harder; by one estimate, the typical rural doctor sees 30 percent more patients than the typical doctor practicing in the city.

➤ Rural doctors charge less than urban doctors, and despite their longer hours, they make less money.

Rural and urban doctors are also different in less measurable ways:

➤ Many people believe that rural medical practice, with its greater personal and professional isolation, attracts a more entrepreneurial type of physician, someone comfortable with doing a little of this and a little of that, a medical jack-of-all-trades.

➤ With fewer nearby colleagues to consult, a rural doctor has to be an independent thinker, able to make difficult patient care decisions alone.

➤ Many people believe that rural doctors are also closer to their patients than doctors in urban areas.

Given these differences, it is not surprising that rural doctors have been more resistant to managed care plans than doctors practicing in urban areas. Where urban doctors are accustomed to managed care plans and know the ropes, rural doctors can find it hard to be accountable to a utilization review manager. Doctors in urban areas are aware of the competition—indeed, they may be sharing an office building. Rural doctors often don't think in those terms. So plans that come to a small town seeking discounts in return for a guaranteed patient base—the typical strategy in urban areas—may get a blank stare from a doctor who already has more patients than he or she can handle.

Mental health professionals are in especially short supply in rural areas. Mental health services can be very important in communities undergoing rapid economic and social changes (more on evaluating a plan's mental health and substance abuse treatment provisions in Chapter 19). For example, the boom-bust cycle common to many communities dependent on mining and oil drilling can leave residents particularly vulnerable to problems involving alcohol, substance abuse, and violence.

> **Your Personal Rx**
> Tell your doctor when you join a managed care plan. Doctors don't know what is happening with their patients unless their patients tell them. Your explanation of your plan and your needs may affect your doctor's decision about his enrollment as a provider.

Mid-Level Professionals

Healthspeak

A *nurse practitioner* is a registered nurse who has completed an advanced training program in primary health care delivery. A *physician assistant* works with or under the supervision of a physician to provide diagnostic or therapeutic care. A *certified nurse-midwife* provides gynecological care and prenatal care; delivers babies; comanages high-risk pregnancies with physicians; and cares for mothers and babies after birth.

While doctors are scarcer in rural areas than in urban areas, many mid-level medical professionals such as *nurse practitioners*, *physician assistants*, and *certified nurse-midwives* are often more willing to live in rural areas. Both urban and rural managed care plans are making increased use of mid-level professionals. Expect rural managed care plans especially to use such professionals, due in part to the difficulty of attracting adequate numbers of doctors to many rural areas.

Remember, mid-level professionals are licensed by the state and do not practice outside their area of competence. Depending on state law, some mid-level practitioners have the authority to prescribe some medications. Some can manage patients independently of physicians but must be able to consult, collaborate with, and refer patients to physicians when appropriate. They can be especially good choices for routine primary care, adult and pediatric, that a rural doctor may be too busy to handle.

Rural Hospitals: Small Can Be Beautiful, but Bigger May Be Better

Hospitals are no longer at the center of care. We are less likely to spend the night in a hospital than we were, say, ten years ago. If you have surgery, chances are it will be at a free-standing surgical center or at the hospital's own outpatient surgical facility.

So what's happening in the hospital? With more outpatient care, hospitals are specializing or realigning the care they give, or closing. Somewhere in the country, a hospital closes—forever—every two weeks.

Rural hospitals are smaller, have even fewer patients, do fewer surgical procedures, and are at greater risk of closing. It is not unusual for a 20-bed hospital to have only two patients. And while practice may not make perfect, it definitely does improve patient outcomes (see Chapter 6 for more on this issue). Managed care companies in a small town or rural area will often bypass small local hospitals in favor of larger, more cost-effective ones further away.

Yet rural areas need more than emergency medical services to ensure adequate access to health care. Some patients will need to be treated by a doctor, not just a paramedic or an emergency medical technician, to ensure their chances of survival and full recovery. To meet these needs and deliver quality care, rural hospitals are gradually being transformed to leaner operations. They stabilize the patient, making sure that she can be moved safely, and then transfer her to larger facilities for further care. The result is that Aunt Jean's foot surgery will not be done at the local hospital but at a specialty center five exits up the interstate.

Sometimes you can feel like the ball in a pinball game. And continuity of care can suffer.

If you belong to a managed care plan that uses hospitals only outside your community, find out how that hospital's *discharge planning department* works. Ask these questions:

➤ Can that department identify the resources in your community—such as home health care, physical therapy, or housekeeping services—that you will need to complete your recovery, or will you be on your own?

➤ Will they pay for those services?

➤ Will your follow-up appointments be scheduled with your regular doctor, or will you have to use a doctor further away?

➤ What should you do if there are complications from your surgery or an emergency? Can you go to your own doctor even if the doctor is not in the network? Are you covered for emergency care if you go to your local hospital?

> **Healthspeak**
> A hospital's *discharge planning department* coordinates the follow-up care and other resources a patient leaving the hospital will need to continue recovering at home.

Special Rules for Specialty Care

Rare diseases and complex medical conditions defy geography. They can happen anywhere. What happens to you, the managed care plan member, when you need—or want—to be seen by a specialist? What happens when your plan doesn't offer a specialist in that field? Specialty care is also important for health problems involving children. Kids are not "small adults"; their needs are different (more on when to see a specialist in Chapters 16 and 17). Even in routine surgery, for example, some doctors recommend using an anesthesiologist with special experience with children.

Let's assume that your plan has agreed to refer you to an appropriate outside specialist (if not, read Chapters 23 and 24). But there's a catch: You (or your child) will need care for a lengthy period of time, but the specialist is located too far away to make commuting practical. Some people literally relocate for as long as the treatment takes. This may be your only option if you are taking part in an experimental protocol or clinical trial; for example, the treatment, by definition, is not available anywhere else (more on experimental treatments in Chapter 18).

In other cases, you may be able to get the treatment you need near your home, but you and your doctor(s) may want expert advice in designing the treatment plan. In the case of a child with cancer, your local community may have adequate facilities for administering radiation and chemotherapy, but your oncologist may welcome advice on the latest techniques and results in treating children.

You may be able to consult a specialist for the design of a treatment plan, which your local doctor would then execute and supervise. You would come back to see the specialist on an occasional basis for progress reports and review.

Your Personal Rx

Make sure your local doctor is actively involved in seeking consulting doctors, when necessary, because he or she would still have the basic responsibility for your care. Competent doctors welcome consultation and input from colleagues. If yours shows a reluctance to seek, or to have you seek, other opinions, change doctors.

Healthspeak

Telemedicine is the use of interactive audio and visual links to enable rural health practitioners to consult in "real time" with specialists in distant medical centers. Applications range from the simple use of the telephone for data transmission to full-motion, two-way interactive video for medical consultation.

The specialist you select could be reluctant to prescribe—and potentially take responsibility for the outcome of—treatment he or she is unable to supervise. The long-distance specialist can't be sure his or her directions are followed exactly or may assume that equipment and techniques are available locally that, in fact, are not. Even simple symptoms that arise in the course of treatment may have a different meaning for a specialist who deals with your condition routinely than for your regular doctor, who may see it less frequently.

If something goes wrong with your care, the distant specialist could face legal liability far out of proportion to his or her actual involvement with your day-to-day care. So both you and your local doctor may have to be especially committed to making a long-distance treatment relationship work. But if all of you are willing to work together and are committed to solving problems before they arise, the use of a consulting specialist can expand the resources available in your plan and your community.

Depending on the resources available in your community, the risks of long-distance specialty care can be reduced—and the benefits increased—by the use of *telemedicine*. Advanced audio and visual techniques can enable the distant doctor to see exactly what your local physician sees, allowing you to save at least some time and travel involved in keeping face-to-face appointments. Find out what telemedicine facilities are available in your community and what your plan's reimbursement policies for such consultations are.

Asking the Right Questions; Getting the Right Answers

Transferred from New York to rural upstate? Leaving Chicago for a new job in the rolling hills downstate? Don't assume that the plan you are being offered covers prescription drugs, eye examinations, or other care that may be important to you, just because it used to offer them when you lived in the city. With fewer providers and potential patients, there will be less competition for patients in rural areas. Rural plans may offer less generous benefit packages or fewer of the extras that can catch the eye of the harried health care coverage shopper.

Be careful when you evaluate quality measures and report cards provided by plans. Various quality measures—such as hospitalization rates for pediatric asthma or five-year breast cancer survival rates—depend on large numbers for validity. In a small community, a given condition may not occur enough times to be measured correctly. If a plan is just entering your community, it may not have a track record there even if the market area is large enough to calculate valid performance measures.

Managed care plans may provide you with quality measures based only on their performance nationwide, in the nearest large urban area, or with your employer's workers in another area. Such data may be useful to you for a general comparison of plans, but the bottom line is that the enrollment material you get from managed care plans may have missing pieces if it doesn't highlight local information. Quality measures that are not calculated for your locality do not take into account the availability and quality of your community's health care resources. If you decide to join a plan based on what the plan and other sources tell you about its quality of care, ask tough questions about duplicating those results in your community.

Don't Keep Your Distance

What happens to you when the managed care bandwagon pulls up to your doctor's door? It depends. If your doctor is able and willing to enroll in your plan, you may be able to continue as if nothing ever happened. But if not, how you get your health care could change dramatically.

A large employer in a rural area may draw employees from many miles around. Some of these employees may live in small cities with a selection of health care providers within a comfortable distance.

But other employees in the same market area may have a harder time using network providers due to longer travel distances. Many plans operating in rural areas have developed innovative techniques for managing care over longer distances.

Coinsurance By the Mile

Network-based plans such as PPOs or POS plans typically establish lower coinsurance rates for care obtained from network providers (the member may pay ten percent of usual and customary charges) than for care obtained outside the network (the member may pay 30 percent). But to take account of the scarcity of rural providers, plans sometimes impose limits on how far their members should be required to travel—8 to 15 miles is common—to consult a network provider. People who live farther from a network provider than this limit can still consult one and receive the plan's best reimbursement rate. But their penalty for using non-network providers will be lower than for those living within the prescribed distance.

Call First

Even plans with few or no providers in a rural community have established ways to manage their members' use of health care. Many plans require that members wanting an appointment with a doctor first explain their problem to an advice nurse on a toll-free hot line. Depending on the problem, the nurse may advise home care, seeing a doctor during regular office hours, or immediate emergency care. Members who first consult the advice nurse receive the plan's preferred coinsurance rate, while those who do not pay a higher rate.

Destination: Retirement!

About one in five rural counties are what the federal government has called *destination retirement* counties. Retired people may move back "home" or simply leave the cities in search of a cheaper and simpler lifestyle.

Healthspeak

A *destination retirement* county is one where at least 15 percent more people age 65 and older are moving in than are moving out.

Seniors who have become accustomed to managed care plans, either during their working careers or after retirement, could have to learn different patterns of health care use in rural areas. Many rural areas do not have HMOs that undertake Medicare contracts. As a result, rural seniors may have to return to traditional Medigap plans or may find they have only one Medicare HMO available that does not offer the attractive benefits often available in large urban areas where the competition is stiffer.

Rural seniors considering a managed care plan should pay special attention to the location of the hospitals the plan requires them to use, the plan's coverage for home health care, and the availability of home health care providers in their communities. Rural residents tend to travel farther than urban residents for most of their needs, anyway, so a healthy senior evaluating a managed care plan may not be concerned about travel distances.

But consider what would happen if you or your spouse were facing a lengthy hospital stay:

➤ Regular visits from friends and family help everybody recover faster, and, indeed, family members may be needed on a regular basis to make decisions about care. Would you or your spouse be able to drive to the hospital frequently?

➤ If you are relocating to a new community or one you left many years ago, are your closest friends and family far away?

➤ Even if you have a network of family and friends in your rural community, do they have the same mobility problems you face?

➤ Home health care can be a great option for people who don't need to be in a full-service hospital but still need care to complete their recovery. Seniors may not "spring back" as quickly from a hospital stay as younger people and may derive particular benefit from professional assistance for a period of time. Is there good quality home health care in your community?

It's an Emergency

Call 911, right?

Wrong!

Many states still don't have statewide "911" systems, meaning that outside urban areas, 911 is a "wrong number." Know what the emergency numbers are for your area and keep them handy. Yes, even on your vacation! Okay, so it sounds a little morbid to arrive in that bucolic vacation cabin and look up the local emergency number even before you unpack your bathing suit or hiking boots. But remember two things:

➤ Vacations are when people do things they do only a few times a year, such as boating, parasailing, and rock climbing. These and other vacation activities are potentially dangerous if you're out of practice, and sometimes, even if you aren't.

➤ In an emergency, calling help directly rather than dialing the operator can save you or your loved ones precious time.

What does all this have to do with managed care? Even when you are on vacation, your plan expects to have a say in your health care. Go where you have to for emergency care, but call once you get there. See Chapter 20 for more tips on staying in touch with your health plan when you are out of town.

The Least You Need to Know

➤ Managed care plans sometimes operate differently in rural areas than in urban areas. Don't assume you know the rules just because you may have used managed care before.

➤ If you need specialty care not available in your community or in your plan, explore creative ways of networking with more distant specialists.

➤ In an emergency, ask to be taken to your nearest hospital. After your condition has been stabilized, you may have to move to a contract hospital under your plan.

➤ Find out if your plan's hospital(s) can coordinate post-hospital care in your community; don't be "home alone."

➤ Don't expect 911 to be wherever you are.

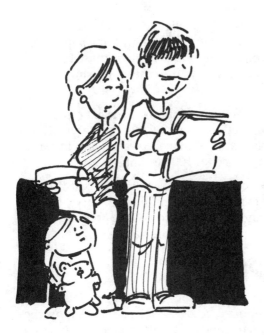

Medicaid

One of the most important problems facing the health care system has been the stubbornly steady share of the population—about one in every six under the age of 65—without health care coverage. If you're not covered, chances are you're more likely to do without needed preventive care, wait longer to see a doctor when you are sick, and be sicker when you do get care than people who have coverage.

Medicaid—the joint state-federal health care coverage program for low-income and sick or disabled people—is the health safety net for some 36 million people who might not otherwise have access to coverage.

Don't pass up this chapter just because you have coverage under an employer plan or a plan you buy on your own. Your elderly parents or grandparents may come under the Medicaid umbrella, as can foster children. Remember, foster children are wards of the

Caution

Foster children who have been placed with you by state or local authorities are not typically eligible for coverage under employer-sponsored health plans. Because such children are wards of the state, however, they are automatically covered under Medicaid, the joint federal-state program for certain low-income individuals and families.

state and thus usually are not eligible for coverage under your employer's health plan (more on this in Chapter 7). Medicaid is also important to the elderly because it is the only public program that pays the costs of nursing-home care.

Most states are now actively adopting managed care for their Medicaid populations. Nationwide, about one in three Medicaid beneficiaries are in managed care plans; in some states, this share approaches 100 percent.

Medicaid enrollees can face both benefits and costs from the expansion of managed care. In this chapter, we tell you what to expect—and what to avoid—as the Medicaid managed care revolution sweeps the nation.

If You've Seen One Medicaid Plan...

If you think private-sector managed care plans are a varied lot, just wait until you see Medicaid managed care plans. The operative number here is 50—as in 50 states (plus the District of Columbia, to be accurate). Medicaid, remember, is a *joint* federal-state program. With Medicaid—as with many other such joint programs—the federal government is like a strict but practical parent. Parents want kids to follow their rules, but most parents with some common sense want their kids to grow up to realize their full adult potential.

In a similar fashion, the federal government sets down guidelines within which the states are to operate their Medicaid programs. But, recognizing that the states differ from each other, the federal government allows states to obtain *waivers* of the federal Medicaid law to test new concepts or approaches to serving their Medicaid populations. Waivers allow each state to do its own thing, so long as it does the equivalent of observing its curfew and putting gas in the family car. Nearly all the states currently have at least one Medicaid waiver on the books.

So please believe us when we say: If you've seen one Medicaid program, you've seen *one* Medicaid program.

House Call

Federal waivers can allow states to require some or all Medicaid beneficiaries to enroll in managed care plans or to implement managed care in only part of the state. Waivers can also allow states to test new ways of administering Medicaid plans, including enrolling beneficiaries in plans that serve mostly Medicaid beneficiaries and extending coverage to low-income individuals and families not eligible for "traditional" Medicaid.

In contrast, think about Medicare, the health care coverage component of the Social Security program (covered in Chapter 8). That program is all federal. From Maine to California, from Washington state to Florida, the same rules apply. Life is simpler that way, though not as varied.

Down the Runway: Medicaid Models

If you or a family member are covered under Medicaid or hope to be, you'll feel more comfortable if you can recognize the major types of managed care plans currently in use under Medicaid. Each type offers you different choices and requires a different mind-set.

Primary Care Case Management

No, this has nothing to do with carrying the doctor's black bag. In a primary care case management system, you have to pick a primary care physician who serves as your gatekeeper into the health care system (more on gatekeepers and their care and feeding in Chapter 11).

Remember, in a gatekeeper system, you go through the gate, or you go nowhere. Either clear everything through the gatekeeper, or you pay for the care yourself. About a third of Medicaid managed care beneficiaries are in gatekeeper-based systems.

HMO

In an HMO, the plan gets a fixed monthly fee to treat you, and you get a comprehensive range of services. That means all the health care you should need is under one roof, subject to the usual warnings about medical necessity (see Chapter 5) and the irresistible impulses of managed care plans to control costs. HMOs account for just under half of Medicaid beneficiaries who are in managed care plans.

Other Prepaid Plans

If you're not in a primary care case management plan or an HMO, you're probably in a prepaid plan that provides a limited range of services. If you want a service the plan does not provide—mental health and substance abuse services are common—you seek it on a fee-for-service basis through traditional Medicaid. Just under one in four Medicaid beneficiaries in managed care plans are covered under this type of arrangement.

Under a plan that provides comprehensive care, someone else (the plan or your gatekeeper doctor) coordinates your health care for you. Coordination can mean nice things, like making sure that your prescriptions don't conflict with each other or that you get the preventive care you need. If you're partly under the prepaid umbrella and partly under fee-for-service care, the coordination burden is on you. Read Chapter 3 and get those three-ring binders in order to organize your health care!

What's in It for You

Despite having health care coverage, Medicaid beneficiaries have not historically had an easy time getting health care. People who became eligible by virtue of low income have often had problems finding doctors and hospitals in the neighborhoods where they live, because low-income areas tend to be underserved.

In addition, since Medicaid limits the amount it pays health care providers to rates that are usually below those in the private market, doctors, even when available, have often not been willing to accept Medicaid patients. Low reimbursement rates can be especially problematic for providers treating people who become eligible for Medicaid by virtue of sickness or disability, because such people tend to be high users of health care.

Finally, even when health care is available and accessible, Medicaid patients may not get as much out of their health care as do other patients. For many Medicaid patients, lack of education or language barriers can complicate compliance with medical regimens, leading to frustration on the part of both doctor and patient. The net result for many Medicaid patients was unmet health care needs coupled with over reliance on hospital emergency rooms for primary care treatment.

Medicaid managed care can redress some of these imbalances for some patients.

➤ Once a Medicaid beneficiary is enrolled in a managed care plan, he or she is free from the need to search around for someone willing to provide treatment at the prices Medicaid is willing to offer. The very act of joining a managed care plan involves "joining" a provider (or group of providers) as well.

➤ Just as for privately insured patients, Medicaid managed care can improve health care coordination. In particular, comprehensive health care coverage plans can provide access to preventive care and early intervention that is particularly important for low-income people or those with chronic health conditions.

➤ The introduction of managed care in some states has been accompanied by benefit improvements for Medicaid patients. For example, in some plans, high-risk maternity patients without home telephones have been issued cellular phones to facilitate access to medical advice.

➤ You may find it easier to enroll in Medicaid managed care than in traditional Medicaid. In particular, many states are separating eligibility for Medicaid managed care from eligibility for Aid to Families with Dependent Children (AFDC), the nation's principal welfare program. So you may not have to be eligible for—or apply for—welfare to enroll in Medicaid managed care.

➤ If you have a foster child, a Medicaid managed care plan could save you trouble in locating a doctor. Many doctors don't participate in the plan because it doesn't pay much, and there are no central lists of those who do participate. Before signing up with a plan, however, find out if its providers are in convenient locations and are accepting new patients.

Don't Let Your Guard Down

But just enrolling in a managed care plan does not eliminate all the concerns Medicaid beneficiaries should have about adequate access to health care. Here are some of the potential problems you should be aware of.

Now You See It, Now You Don't: The Vanishing Health Care System

Some managed care plans don't contract with health care providers who have taken care of Medicaid populations. This refusal can make it harder for beneficiaries to get care, since they would no longer be reimbursed for care obtained from the providers they were used to using. The new doctors, clinics, or hospitals may be better than what you, the beneficiary, had before, but if you have to travel inordinate distances, or if the new providers are not accessible by public transportation, you may not get the care you need when you need it. Likewise, if the plan refuses to enroll your doctor because he or she cannot meet board certification requirements, you may find health care harder to get than before managed care made it "easier."

> **Your Personal Rx**
> If your plan's choice of doctors, location of facilities, or other organizational decisions make it hard for you to get care, your plan may be in violation of federal anti-discrimination statutes. Raise the question with your plan's member services department; you may be glad you did! Some plans whose location or contracting decisions have been challenged on these grounds have instituted or expanded free transportation for their members to their facilities.

Starting Up Is Hard to Do

If you're a Medicaid beneficiary who is not already in a managed care plan, your turn may not be far off. Be forewarned: The transition from traditional medicine to managed care may not be smooth when it happens. Some states have not allowed enough time to put managed care in place, with confusion the inevitable result.

There's not much you can do if the whole system is off track except keep asking questions—about your plan, new-member materials, your new providers—until you are satisfied with the answers. And be sure to keep Chapter 3 handy when you do!

> **House Call**
> States receive Medicaid waivers from the federal government for two to five years at a time, depending on the type of waiver. If you have problems with your plan, and make them known, your state's program could be redesigned the next time it comes up for renewal. See Chapter 25 for where to take your complaints.

Beware of Direct Marketing

If you answer your door to find a health care plan representative with a turkey, don't start the oven just yet. Door-to-door marketing of managed care plans to Medicaid beneficiaries has been characterized by some—literally—ham-handed tactics. Indeed, many states have banned direct and door-to-door marketing by these plans entirely. When you choose your plan, do so on the basis of hard information—not dinner.

Your Personal Rx

If you have trouble getting your plan's list of providers—before or after choosing a plan—or are not permitted to choose your provider, complain to your state's department of social services, to the federal government, or both (see Chapter 25). Your access to the health care you need when you need it could be at stake.

Informed Consumer? They May Not Make It Easy

One of the best tools you can use to select the right health care plan for you is the plan's list of health care providers (see Chapter 6 for more on this). But that's only if you can get it. Some Medicaid managed care beneficiaries may not get a list of providers until *after* they have selected a plan—if at all. The fault may lie with the state; many states do not require plans to make their provider lists available to beneficiaries before they must select a plan.

And it can get worse. You may not even be allowed to select your own provider! Instead, you could be arbitrarily assigned to a provider the plan selects for you.

Separate but Equal? Maybe...

You say you see ads for managed care plans on the bus or TV but can't find the plans on your Medicaid list? Don't be surprised. Many Medicaid managed care beneficiaries are enrolled in Medicaid-only plans.

Sometimes this happens for entirely appropriate reasons. For example, in some states, providers who had traditionally treated low-income patients formed their own managed care plans when their state's Medicaid program turned to managed care. Such plans would allow Medicaid beneficiaries to continue to use their previous providers. New plans may also need to be formed to serve people in areas without enough providers.

Sometimes the reasons are less benign. In some states that have turned to Medicaid managed care, commercial managed care plans have not had the capacity to enter the Medicaid market or have been uninterested for other reasons. Or a commercial plan may contract with Medicaid but only make part of its network available to the Medicaid beneficiaries it enrolls.

Whether "separate" can *ever* be "equal" in health care is beyond the scope of this book to decide. But if your plan takes an inordinately long time to schedule an appointment, to refer you for specialty care, or to respond to a complaint, make your voice heard. Unless you've been caught up in start-up problems—which should correct themselves—you may be getting substandard service, and ultimately, care.

Rules, Rules, Rules

Some managed care plans have procedures and requirements that may not work in a Medicaid setting. For example, it's not uncommon for plans to require that all appointments be made by telephone. But what if you don't have one? Or what if you have one but can't understand the language spoken by the person at the other end of the line?

Don't be shut out. We hate to sound like a broken record, but make your concerns known to the plan's member services department, your state or local department of social services, or both. It usually won't take an act of Congress to make exceptions to onerous rules such as requiring that all appointments be made by phone. And unless you speak up, people who make such decisions may not even know there is a problem.

Your Personal Rx
If you can't get your problems addressed either by your plan or by your state or local department of social services, vote with your feet if you can. If you are offered a choice of plans and leave one that is unresponsive to your needs, trust us, people will notice.

The Least You Need to Know

➤ Many states are using Medicaid to extend health care coverage to people who don't have a foothold in the private system. Even if you're working, if you don't have coverage (or a lot of money!), check with your state or local department of social services to see if you're eligible for coverage.

➤ If you move, even within the same state, your health care coverage options could change. Check with the department of social services in your new community to see what might be available for you.

➤ Medicaid managed care plans differ significantly in structure. In some states, you may have one foot in traditional coverage and one in managed care; make sure you know which foot is where.

➤ Some Medicaid managed care plans have been implemented in a hurry. Make sure you ask enough questions to know the rules—as well as your rights.

➤ Managed care can correct some of the problems that Medicaid beneficiaries have historically faced in obtaining care. But it can also create new ones. Insist on your right to choose a plan and a provider, and to get timely service. If your managed care plan is short-changing you, you may have recourse under civil rights laws.

Part 3
Using Your Plan

Okay, you've picked your plan, and you think you've made a pretty good choice. Now how do you make the best use of your plan from day to day? How do you get your money's worth—and stay healthy at the same time?

To do this, you need to understand the basic elements of the health care system. These include primary care, preventive care, and emergency care. Primary care is what you need when either your health problem is pretty routine or when you don't know what you have and you want someone to point you in the right direction. Preventive care is what you need to stay healthy and to find any problems that arise while they are still easy to deal with. Emergency care is—you think you know this one, don't you?—harder to define than you may think from watching medical shows on TV.

And we have found that men and women use health care very differently; that is, women use it, and men try their best to avoid it. So in this section, we look at the health care system from both the male and the female points of view.

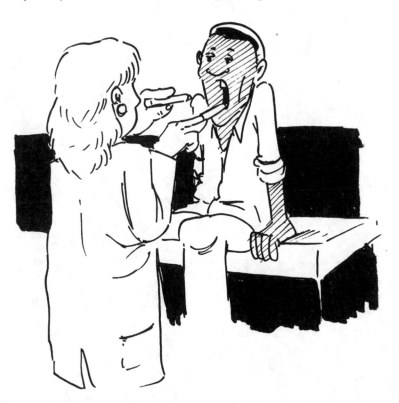

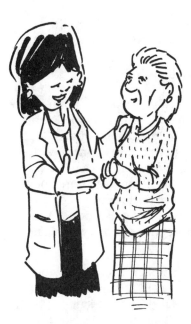

Chapter 11

Primary Care: The Gateway to Health Care

In This Chapter

➤ Getting a good primary care physician

➤ How to pick and use a pediatrician

➤ The wrong choice: if you don't like your doctor

➤ Working at the relationship

Your primary care doctor is the general contractor for your body, and sometimes your mind. She is the one who understands how the various treatments you are receiving fit together—or don't. She is the one who monitors your prescription drug interactions, overall health, and preventive care. But these general contractors may also be the guards at the entrance to more medical care from your health plan. Their role as "gatekeeper" to the larger health care system is part of the foundation upon which managed care is built. Their stature (and sometimes their salaries) is growing, as they take on the responsibilities of referrals and day-to-day management of some chronic diseases. He coordinates testing and sometimes acts as the translator between you and the specialist. The primary care doctor can also be involved in mental health services.

If you want to retain some control over your care, get a primary care doctor with whom you can work. In many plans, he has the keys to treatment, so it's imperative you chose one who can treat, refer, and communicate with you effectively.

This chapter gives you information on what primary care doctors do, why they are important, and how to work with them to get the best care your plan can give.

Introducing Your Primary Care Physician

Your doctor is primary because he provides basic or general health care at the point where you first seek assistance from the medical system. He is also your chief, or main, doctor. Your primary care doctor is a family, general practice doctor or internist for you, or a pediatrician for your children. (See Chapter 13 for when ob/gyn's can be primary care physicians.) Your primary care doctor is not only the one you go to for your flu, strep throats, and physicals, but also your primary coordinator of care if you need someone other than a primary care doctor. In an HMO, your primary care doctor can arrange for hospital admissions. Primary care doctors are the overlords of the referral process. And the primary care doctor can be an advocate for you and ensure the continuity of medical records for timely communications among the "health team."

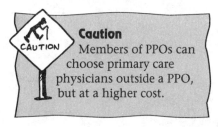

Caution
Members of PPOs can choose primary care physicians outside a PPO, but at a higher cost.

What primary care doctors do is something of a moving target. For years, they were defined in the same terms as other medical specialties—by a label. Here's a surgeon, here's a neurosurgeon, and here's a neurologist. Now they are defined by their functions. Those functions stress relationships and collaborations rather than boundaries among specialists. They manage a health problem in a large system so that the patient knows who is directing and coordinating her care. They can be advocates in a large system, and they can ensure the continuity of medical records for timely communications among the "health team."

That is, in a perfect world.

If your primary care doctor doesn't deliver the goods, you can have real problems. So pick a good one. The following section is designed to help you do just that.

Finding Your Perfect Match

Where do you start? Start with your plan's list of physicians. For a list of the plan's primary care doctors, call your member services department. They will mail you a list.

Even if your plan is a very good one, choosing just any primary care doctor from its list doesn't do the trick. You have to find the doctor who is right for you, who meets your needs, and with whom you can talk.

Lose the "doctor is my friend" mentality. The Marcus Welby School of Medicine is folklore at best. Great friends sometimes practice terrible medicine. The "partnership" aspect stressed by managed care plans is also suspect, because you and your plan are not at an equal level of power. We think a better benchmark to use is "treat me like an adult." You want to be able to make decisions about your health with all the information available. Any questions *you* deem important must be answered to *your* satisfaction, and treatment decisions made with all the pertinent facts made available to you.

The List: What to Look for in a Primary Care Doctor

We've put together a list to use when choosing a primary care doctor. Some of these considerations may be more important to you than others, and some may not figure into your calculations at all because of your own circumstances. So consider them all, and then choose the ones most useful to you:

Your Personal Rx

Don't wait for a sick day to pick a primary care physician. When you change plans, make finding your primary care doctor and pediatrician a first priority. Ask your new plan about its policy for getting records from the previous plan. Schedule everyone in your family for a visit during the first month so you are established with a doctor.

➤ Ask friends and family about the doctors you're considering. If they've used them in the past, they may be good judges of how easy it is to talk to the doctor and how long it takes to get an appointment.

➤ Check out the doctor's credentials. You can ask the plan's and the doctor's office for information on his training and experience. Ask your plan about board certification, including when the doctor was last certified. Also check out any local surveys on physicians and plans. (See Chapter 6 for information on surveys.)

House Call

The American Medical Association has Physician Select, a free Internet service for information on physicians (**http://www.ama-assn.org**). Public Citizen's Health Research Group, a public interest group in Washington, D.C., publishes *13,012 Questionable Doctors*, containing the names of doctors who continue to practice medicine despite records of incompetence and other problems. It is updated every three years. Call 1-800-289-3787 to order a copy, or check your local library.

➤ Can you get there? Do you want to keep your entire family's care close to home, or would you prefer it be close to your office? If you are continuing with a certain specialist, is there a primary care doctor you could use in his building?

Your Personal Rx

When you check out location, also ask how long it takes for routine exams and the basic sick visit. Also find out from your health plan if lab tests are done at the doctor's office and, if not, where they are done. Knowing how long and where you need to go helps evaluate the location.

➤ Do the office hours start early? Does the doctor have appointments after 5 p.m.? Are there Saturday hours? Does she make home visits? If you have to rearrange heaven and earth to get there on time, this is not the doctor for you.

➤ Some tips apply to choosing just about everything from restaurants to day care centers. Is the doctor's office orderly and clean? Does the staff seem honest and respectful? Do the doctor and the office staff appear sober? Physicians can have trouble with alcohol or substance abuse, too.

➤ Are patient records scattered about in the open, or have they taken care to keep them private? Your doctor and office staff should care about confidentiality as much as you do.

➤ If the whole office belongs to your plan, assess the other doctors in the practice. You may have to use one if your doctor is not available. Do you have a choice between appointments with the nurse practitioner and the doctor? Some patients prefer the doctor only, while others prefer the nurse practitioner, and others don't really care.

House Call

HMOs are more likely than other forms of managed care to use physician assistants and nurse practitioners. Good nonphysician providers (as they are called in managed care lingo) can be very good at delivering primary care, health maintenance, and health promotion activities, and tend to spend more time with patients.

➤ Can you get an answer from the doctor late at night? Most doctors use an answering service and the doctor on duty calls back. Sometimes even the nurse-practitioner is on duty. Many managed care plans have an advice line answered 24 hours a day, usually by registered nurses. It can help you decide whether you need to come in for urgent care or can just be a comfort during those exhausting, late-night bouts with a fever or stomach flu.

➤ If you have a chronic condition, you will still need a primary care doctor. Ask if she has experience with your condition and how she manages it. Find out if the plan or practice has a primary care doctor who is an expert in your condition. For example, one company persuaded their HMO to take on a primary care doctor who was an expert in HIV treatment. They felt he would know when to refer in situations that a garden-variety primary care doctor would not necessarily know.

➤ Have a frank discussion about referrals with your doctor, especially if you have a chronic condition. Ask him about how he makes that decision. Find out from the doctor and the plan if you can get referrals by phone.

➤ Find out how familiar he is with managed care or your plan. Ask, "How long have you been with this health plan? What is your experience with managed care organizations generally?" Get an idea if he knows how to operate in the bureaucracy.

One of the ways to check out the doctor is to see if you can get an interview appointment. That may be your physical, which means you have to choose the doctor first and ask questions later. If you have a chronic condition, it may be worthwhile to pay for that interview.

Is It a Good Fit?

You and your doctor need to know each other really well from the beginning. When you interview your new doctor, ask how much experience she has with your type of patient (that is, chronic condition, high pain threshold, fearful, and so on). Is he open to treatments that don't rely heavily on medication (if that is important to you)? What preventive programs does he suggest to someone like you (age, sex, health status)? The answers to these questions will help him understand the type of patient you are and help you understand what to expect of him.

Now balance your needs. You've gotten the information on training, location, and the doctor's opinions about treatment, but is it a good fit? Do you feel at ease enough to tell her about yourself or your family? For instance, you have three kids, ages 10, 14, and 16. You are looking at two pediatricians, one 1 mile away and one 2.5 miles away. The one 2.5 miles away has special training in adolescent medicine. That doctor might be a good bet. However, if you and your kids feel most comfortable with the one closer, go for it.

If you are in a Medicare HMO, you should be especially concerned about how many doctors are accepting new patients and how long you have to wait for an appointment. People over age 65 use increasingly more medical services, so your chances of getting an appointment may suffer if the plan hasn't kept up with an increasing Medicare enrollment.

Also ask about the plan's use of physician assistants and nurse practitioners. It may use them to offset the increased demand. If you are comfortable with them, it may ease your mind. If you are not, you should know who will deliver your care.

Finally, focus on the whole picture: the doctor and her staff. Getting good care relies on good relationships among you, the doctor, her nurses or nurse practitioners, and office staff. They are often the ones who have to take on the bureaucracy of the managed care plan to get you the care you need.

119

Where's My Referral? Primary Doctors as Gatekeepers

The gatekeeper's duties are exactly what you would expect them to be. Before going through the gates of managed care to more medical care, you have to get the gatekeeper to let you in. Most often, that gatekeeper is your primary care doctor, who is the one responsible for referring you to other doctors.

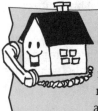

House Call

Doctors feel the health plan's judgment on referrals. Many view the reason that doctors are dropped by plans is because of too many referrals or tests, rather than bad practices. "The referral comparison is always before us," said one family practitioner.

A referral is the okay from your primary care doctor for you to see a specialist. Sometimes it's the okay from the specialist to see a subspecialist (more on this in Chapter 16). If you are in an HMO, you must get one before you go on to the specialist, or you go at your financial peril. If you are in a PPO, you may be able to go through the gates without the stop at the primary care doctor, or you may have to check in with the gatekeeper, too.

But there are exceptions: Some plans allow (and some states require) direct access that allows you to go to a specific type of doctor without checking in with your primary care doctor (or in spite of checking in with your primary care doctor). And although direct access allows you to go to some doctors without referrals, that doesn't make the specialist your primary care doctor. You can't go to an ob-gyn if you have conjunctivitis.

Healthspeak

Direct access means you can go to another doctor without having to first go to your primary care doctor (or get a referral), either by law or as allowed by the plan. Obstetrics and gynecology are the most common specialties to have direct access, but there are others. For example, Georgia allows direct access for dermatologists, Arkansas for eye care providers, and Kentucky for chiropractors.

Here are some tips for working with your primary care doctor to ease a process that can make your (and your doctor's) life miserable.

Respect the referral process. Keep track of your referrals. They are important pieces of paper. Most referrals in HMOs are for a specific number of visits or length of time. After that, you have to go back to see your primary care doctor. Make sure you know when you have to check back. Patients in plans that require written referrals also often ask doctors to post-date referrals if they went to a specialist without getting prior approval. This is a no-no. Doctors are sometimes fined for this by the plan.

Many primary care doctors asked us to emphasize their role as coordinator of care and how important it is in a managed care setting. A referral to the specialist is often for consultation only, with the treatment staying with the primary care doctor. If it goes beyond consultation, it is the "special" part that is transferred to the specialist; the rest of the patient's care stays with the primary care doctor.

Special Considerations for Pediatricians

If you have small children, you may spend as much time at the pediatrician's office as at the grocery store. Even that 14-year-old who is six inches taller and 30 pounds heavier than you can expect to spend considerable time there with various physicals, ailments, and adolescent-only problems.

In some ways, pediatricians treat the whole family. They get to know everyone's histories, styles of coping, and personalities. When you switch plans (necessitating a switch of pediatricians), this "intangible" knowledge is lost. Put this into the mix when you are considering changing plans, especially if your kids are adolescents. If your teenager is comfortable with her pediatrician, you may want to stay with that practice during the "turbulent" years. Trusting the doctor at this age is very important for communication and treatment.

Choosing Your Pediatrician

If you are required to change pediatricians, or if you're choosing one for the first time, we have a list of considerations for you. Earlier in this chapter we gave you a list of tips for choosing your primary care doctor. All of those apply to picking a pediatrician, but we've also added a number of other factors:

➤ Communication is on our primary care pick list, but it's even more important when choosing a pediatrician. Given the large number of patients pediatricians see each day, the frequency of your visits, and the emotional charge of having a sick child, the communication has to be open, direct, and aimed at the adult in you.

➤ You will need to call your pediatrician as often as you go to him—maybe more. Find out if 24-hour consultation is available. This may be the advice line for your health plan, or it may be separate. In any case, 24-hour access to consultation is extremely helpful, especially when you're up with a kid with the chicken pox.

➤ Check out the pediatrician's board certification and recertification. You can also ask if the pediatrician teaches medical students or leads conferences at a pediatric hospital. Ask about the types of continuing medical education courses she attends.

➤ Nurse practitioners can be very important to pediatric practices. They can take more time with patient education and developmental exams. Check out if the doctor is supportive of the nurse practitioner. If you have friends or family who use that pediatric practice, ask them how the nurse practitioner is used.

➤ If your child has a chronic condition, talk to the pediatrician about referrals to pediatric specialists. Plans have been known to limit referrals to a few specialists who may not be trained in pediatrics. Check out the pediatrician's knowledge and experience with your child's condition and the specialists to whom he refers (more on this in Chapter 16).

➤ Sick kids and travel always seem to go together. Ask who to contact and what to do if your kids get sick while traveling (as they inevitably do). Double-check with your plan.

The Care and Feeding of Your Pediatrician

You may have to change some of your expectations of what your pediatric visits will be like. One pediatrician in a large, regional HMO told us that the big change in the practice of pediatrics is that patients have more responsibilities. "Managed care has added more responsibility to my patients than to me," she said.

Managed care puts time pressures on busy practices. If you want answers to the myriad questions about your child's health that constantly crop up, you have to be the one to "manage" the communications.

When you call for a sick appointment, mention anything else that needs attention now. If you spring other issues without any notice, it will lead to the "Oh, by the way" visits that doctors dread. A local pediatrician told us that 75 percent of the sick visits also cover, by discussion or exam, one or two more problems than the parent mentioned when they made the appointment. If you don't tell the office staff what you need when you call, and it's not life- or limb-threatening, you could be asked to schedule another appointment.

Your Personal Rx

Many pediatricians told us that sick kids brought by baby-sitters and teenagers alone are problems. The caretakers are often un-informed about health plans and can't adequately explain symptoms. If tests are required, parental per-mission may be needed. Make sure you have an adequate plan for sick visits when you can't be there.

You may be used to having lab work and tests done at your pediatrician's office. Your new plan, or a change in your old plan, may require you to go to labs or facilities under contract to the plan. Check this out when you join the plan. If you suddenly discover during a sick visit that you must take your sick child to a lab five miles away, the inconvenience, added to your mood after two sleepless nights, can lead to a pretty volatile situation.

Pediatric physicals cover lots of ground, including development, growth, and nutrition. When you call for a physical and there are other things on your mind, let the doctor know about it. At the time you make the call, you will be told whether it can be assessed at the time of the physical or if it will require another visit.

Remember how you learned to use medical care at an early age? Use pediatric care to instruct kids on how to handle the managed care system:

➤ Engage them, especially your adolescents. They can prepare their own questions ahead of time, call the doctor's office for appointments, use the urgent care line, and seek information about medications and instructions.

➤ Get them conscious of things like screenings and self-exams. Your pediatrician can be helpful when the "big guys" make the transition from child to adult health.

The Wrong Choice: If You Don't Like Your Doctor

Your plan handbook will have a specific section on choosing your primary care physician. It may also have a section on how to change your primary care doctor. Some plans have limits on how often you can change primary care doctors in a year. You must let member services know about the change, or you could be billed for services or have your claims denied.

If you change doctors within a staff model HMO in one location, your records will not have to be transferred. If you change doctors in another type of plan, it may take two weeks or more to get your records changed.

> **Your Personal Rx**
> Make sure you check your member handbook for any procedures your plan has for changing primary care doctors. Once you make a change, double-check with member services to make sure it is "in the system." It will save you a month of phone calls if you do it right.

Working at the Relationship

Earlier in this chapter, we told you to evaluate potential primary care doctors in much the same way you would evaluate somebody selling any other (expensive) service. We're not changing that advice. But modern medicine, and especially the world of managed care, is full of forces that can drive you and your doctor apart. If you let them, your care will suffer.

Both tight networks such as group and staff model HMOs and loose ones such as PPOs and POS plans can give short shrift to this relationship. You may be in a group model HMO that values health care access and responsiveness to patient concerns. If you call for a same-day appointment, you may get an appointment with the health care provider available when you can make it, rather than the one you have chosen to be responsible for your health.

You're happy because your *immediate* need has been met, but you have lost an important chance to cement your relationship with your primary care physician. If you can, wait or reorganize your schedule so that you can see *your* physician.

If you are in a looser network plan, with few or no constraints on whom you may see, your overall care may suffer because your primary care doctor doesn't know what you are

Your Personal Rx

If you are in a PPO or POS plan, let your primary care doctor know who else you are seeing. Even better, if you are thinking of consulting a specialist, ask your doctor whether you should. He or she may be able to treat your condition as well or better.

doing. Many specialists are careful to send reports back to your primary care doctor, but everybody's busy these days, and paperwork can fall through the cracks. Ask that the reports be sent, alert your primary care doctor's office to ask, or both.

Communication is a two-way street. One of patients' biggest complaints about managed care is short visits with their doctor. Managed care stresses your partnership with them. But you are a participant. One of the ways you participate is by doing your part to make the most of the limited time with your doctor.

Managed care has put time management at the top of your doctor's list of skills. When you make the appointment, tell them what it's about. That way they can say, "Well, I'll need extra time to deal with this."

If you have a nagging rumbling in the tummy that is worrying you, come to your appointment with a list of symptoms and questions. What they are, when they started, what makes them worse, what makes them better, and if you take medications, what effect they have.

Talk symptoms, not diagnosis. Don't say "I'm a mess"; she doesn't know what that means to you personally. It may mean, "I'm not operating at 100 percent of myself," or it may mean, "I can't sleep, eat, exercise, and I have a rash." Don't make your doctor guess; tell her!

Write down what you've been experiencing. You are less likely to forget something and more likely to remember the answers. If you miss what your doctor is saying, ask her to repeat it.

What happens if you have more questions and you are running out of time? Ask anyway. If you come prepared, a good doctor will stick around and answer them. He may suggest a follow-up visit or phone time. If you don't ask, you won't get all the answers you want, and your doctor won't really know what is going on. If your doctor brushes you off without arranging a way to answer those questions, brush her off and find another doctor.

Do you need help keeping track of what your doctor says? Take notes and date them. Take another person along to help remember and ask questions. Take a tape recorder along and tape your conversation. Some doctors recoil from this, but, especially if you might get bad news, your emotional state may edit what you truly hear and remember.

Ask about any drugs your doctor prescribes. What will they do? What side effects can you expect (see also Chapter 16)?

Good communication can go a long way to getting good care in managed care. But it can't go all the way. There are plans that restrict services substantially and go only for the bucks, while giving quality short shrift. The informed consumer also watches his back. If you feel you've done all you can and are still not happy, see Chapters 23, 24, and 25.

The Least You Need to Know

➤ Your choice of primary care physician is one of the most important choices you make in a managed care plan.

➤ Your primary care doctor is responsible for your total care and may be the gatekeeper to more medical care in your plan. Choose one with whom you can talk, and assess his practice and qualifications carefully.

➤ Know your plan's requirements for referrals. Check back with your primary care doctor when your referrals run out.

➤ Pick a pediatrician as though you will go to her for the next 18 years. If you are faced with changing plans, your pediatrician's participation may be a deciding factor.

➤ Take charge of communications between your primary care doctor and yourself. Time pressures can be stringent, so do the most you can to make the most of your time.

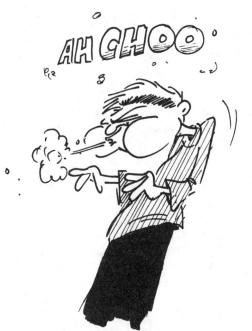

Chapter 12

Preventive Care

In This Chapter

➤ Learning what preventive care is available

➤ Why your HMO stays in touch

➤ Using preventive care to your advantage

➤ What to expect from a physical

➤ When your screening means more tests

➤ Milestones for kids and adults

Pssssst. Want to know what HMOs are good at? Preventive care. After all the talk of services you might not get, rules you have to follow (or else), and how to be your own advocate, this chapter might be a relief. It's the good news side.

But this is today's health care system, so expect it to be more complicated than at first glance. Your alter ego, the Informed Consumer, will once again be in demand. Doesn't that guy ever get a rest? Not while you have to deal with your health care.

Preventive care services are provided to infants and children, adolescents, and adults. They include:

➤ *Screening.* Screening includes periodic physical examinations and laboratory tests based on your medical history and risk assessment, such as family history, smoking, and exercise habits.

➤ *Counseling.* Your primary care doctor or other medical professional explains the relationships between risk factors and health. Through counseling, the health plan assists patients in getting the knowledge, skills, and motivation to adopt and maintain healthy behavior.

➤ *Immunization* and *chemoprophylaxis.* These are vaccinations against infectious diseases and medication to prevent future diseases.

Preventive care is "mass" medicine at its best. Preventive programs are put together to make available services that are demonstrated scientifically to be effective to the population at large (or large groups in the population). That's how preventive care trickles down to you.

House Call

Think of preventive care as a screening, vaccine, or lab test that is as useful to you as to a neighbor, another person your age in the next town, and another person in next state. Preventive care is useful to a large group of people in very broad categories, such as age or gender.

This chapter will tell you about preventive care, what it is and isn't, when to use it, what to expect, and how it fits into your managed care plan.

How Your Plan Chooses What to Do

Notice we said "HMOs" at the beginning of this chapter. All through this book we refer to "managed care," which includes HMOs along with other forms of health care plans. Here we say HMO because that's what we mean. HMOs are at the top of the food chain in preventive care. It's part of their history and their organization. Staff and group model HMOs have more of their own organizations devoted to making decisions about and delivering preventive care than do other types of managed care plans.

Managed care plans focus on guidelines and do not recommend screening outside those groups that meet the "mass" medicine standard. Making the decision to offer a medical screening test to thousands, sometimes millions, of members is a difficult decision. The goal of screening is to test people for diseases that are at such an early stage, or preclinical, that they have yet to produce symptoms. But what do you do with the information? Does knowing it allow you to live longer or catch a disease earlier?

In part, HMOs use national guidelines to help them decide which preventive services to offer. The U.S. Preventive Services Task Force of ten doctors and scientists updated its recommendations in 1996. It reviewed more than 200 diagnostic tests and found many of them ineffective for most people. Its recommendations are in *The Guide to Clinical Preventive Services*, which lists by age and sex the preventive services that are needed. This guide is the gold standard. If you can find a copy in your library, you can use it to look up the tests recommended for you your age and sex and ask your plan and doctor about them.

Your Personal Rx
You can rank managed care plans in terms of their availability of preventive care services: (1) staff or group model HMOs; (2) IPAs; (3) PPOs; and (4) fee-for-service plans. There are variations among HMOs in the preventive care services they offer but much more variation among other types of plans (more on this in Chapter 5). If these services are important to you, enroll in an HMO.

HMOs also set up their own clinical guidelines for preventive services. These are evidence-based, which means that they are the product of a comprehensive search and review of the medical literature rather than a few guys in a room who think that's the way it should be done. HMOs have physicians who design and manage disease prevention and health promotion programs and evaluate their quality and effectiveness.

Specialist organizations and disease groups may also have their own guidelines, many of which are adopted by HMOs. For instance, below are the American Academy of Pediatricians' recommendations for preventive care:

➤ Medical history taken during an initial visit and updated at various times

➤ Height and weight measurements taken during regular office visits

➤ A developmental and behavioral assessment

➤ A thorough physical examination

➤ Guidance on injury prevention

➤ Vision and hearing tested periodically, more frequently if required by a child's individual history

➤ Head circumference measured through 24 months of age

Caution
A diagnostic test not needed by the vast majority of the population may still be appropriate for you. Medical history, family history, and risk factors make certain diagnostic tests more useful for certain people than for the general population. If your history or risk factors deviate from the general population, ask your doctor about the test and why he is for or against it.

- ➤ Immunizations for newborns and at various intervals during infancy and childhood up to age 11
- ➤ Dental referral at age 3
- ➤ Regular blood pressure screening at age 3
- ➤ Lead screening at 9 and 24 months
- ➤ Blood test for hematocrit or hemoglobin levels at around 9 months and age 15
- ➤ Urinalysis at ages 5 and 15
- ➤ Test for sexually transmitted diseases for sexually active adolescents
- ➤ Pelvic exams for sexually active females
- ➤ Screening for tuberculosis
- ➤ Cholesterol screening for high-risk patients or if family history is unavailable

The Messenger and the Message

How do HMOs make you want preventive services? Publicity. Their newsletters and special publications highlight preventive services offered and who should get them.

HMOs are becoming very proficient as "messengers" for preventive care. They have the business support and the administrative capabilities to get out mass mailings and newsletters, even personalized letters to certain groups, such as the elderly or parents of newborns. HMOs can also identify the particular health risks and problems of its member population and develop strategies to deal with them. This might include outreach to patients, chart reminders and other techniques to help deliver preventive services, and health-education and risk-reduction programs.

So if you get a letter addressed to you in the familiar way of an old friend suggesting that you have a mammogram, enter a cholesterol screening program, or even letting you know about a new diet workshop, and it's from someone named "Barbie" at your HMO, you are receiving the outreach part of preventive services.

What does the HMO get out of all this effort? It gets increased patient satisfaction. It may also get overall better patient outcomes and reduce the number of patient visits. It also gets bonus points for quality. The National Committee for Quality Assurance considers a number of preventive services as its quality indicators (for more on quality indicators and HEDIS data, see Chapter 6). These include vaccination rates, mammography, cervical cancer screening, and retinal exams for diabetics. As employers begin to include quality along with price when they make decisions on which plans to offer, they use HEDIS data more. So preventive services become part of the equation when employers look for quality in plans.

Use Preventive Care to Your Advantage

Maybe you simply don't want to go to the doctor when you don't have to. Get rid of that thought. The best time to get preventive care is with periodic health exams. And if you used to avoid preventive care because it was expensive, you no longer have an excuse: If you belong to an HMO (or certain other plans), it is already paid for. Remember, the premise of preventive care is that if you get care early, you can stay healthier for longer.

House Call

Some PPOs cover some preventive care, and others set a dollar limit, such as $300 of preventive care. If employers are interested, they can sometimes negotiate more preventive care in their benefit packages.

If you are shopping around for a plan, take a look at whether there are any copayments or deductibles attached to preventive services. Pick a plan without them: Copayments and deductibles can act as disincentives to using services.

Ask your plan for information about its recommended preventive services:

➤ One of the first places you can get a sense of what preventive care you're entitled to is in your member handbook. You can work out a schedule on when to use the preventive care available to you.

➤ Many of the large HMOs have this information on their Websites.

➤ Your plan's monthly newsletters also provide information on preventive care, such as changes in immunization schedules for children (if boosters for measles are recommended, hepatitis shots for teenagers, and so on), and health screening schedules, such as mammograms or vision tests.

It helps the doctor if you can keep track of services needed and available through your plan. Doctors may belong to lots of plans, each with somewhat different preventive services. These services are usually listed in your handbook, so bring it along for reference.

House Call

Preventive care is probably one of the least emphasized areas of medical training. Usually it's a topic required throughout medical education; but to what extent is a different story. It may be a course or a part of a number of courses. Doctors receive their training in hospitals that deal with the sick and the dying, not those who want to stay well.

131

What to Expect from Your Periodic Physical

When you have your annual physical...

Strike that. If you fit within the normal health range for your age and sex, you probably don't need an annual physical, and your plan isn't trying to skimp on you if it doesn't offer it. Studies have found that for most people between the ages of 25 and 64, annual physicals are not necessary.

If you do get a periodic physical, it should consist of age- and sex-specific screenings, focused histories that include risk factors, limited tests, and immunizations as needed. But don't expect a battery of tests unless your basic exam and history tag you as someone who needs further testing.

If you are still feeling cheated because you think you haven't had enough tests, think again. Preventive care can be given at any time. For instance, if your child is behind on immunizations but is at the doctor for an infected toe, she may catch up on the immunizations then. The emphasis is on getting it to you when you are available, rather than delivering it all at once.

Though there is a lot of information in the popular press about what screenings to get and when for the general population, there have been many conflicting reports on who needs what type of testing at what age. The following gives you examples of how this may vary by age:

➤ *Cervical Cancer.* Pap smears should be repeated at least every three years, but may be discontinued after age 65 if they have been consistently normal.

➤ *Prostate Cancer.* The American Cancer Society recommends annual routine screening by digital rectal exam and a blood test called PSA (prostate-specific antigen) for men age 50 and older.

➤ *Cholesterol.* Periodic screening for men 35 to 65 and women 45 to 65. Unless patients show symptoms of heart disease (or family history), the tests are not recommended for children, adolescents, or young adults.

Certain services, such as pap smears, mammography, and some screenings (diabetes, high blood pressure, and others), should be provided more often for high-risk individuals. Those individuals should receive counseling, which may require more visits. Counseling is focused on individual situations that need more frequent reinforcement.

What if, after your exam or screenings, the doctor suggests more frequent screening or further testing? It's time to get educated and ask questions. Tests and screenings are not necessarily risk-free or fail-safe. Find out whether, and how much, a plan pays for a retest, if one is required. Find out whether copayments and deductibles apply to further tests so you're prepared. Check on whether referrals are necessary or whether a primary care doctor or pediatrician is the best one to perform the tests and counsel you.

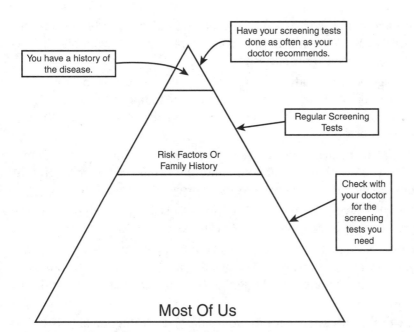

When should you get screening tests?

You have a history of the disease.

Have your screening tests done as often as your doctor recommends.

Regular Screening Tests

Risk Factors Or Family History

Check with your doctor for the screening tests you need

Most Of Us

Use Your Milestones to Ensure Good Health

Managed care—and modern medicine, for that matter—requires you to do more for yourself than your parents might have had to do for themselves. But we wrote this book to help you, not overwhelm you.

You can simplify your health care by making preventive care part of your life, like the way you check the batteries in your smoke detector when you change your clocks in the spring and the fall (you *do* do that, don't you?). Simply add health care to the major changes and milestones in your life and that of your family:

Your Personal Rx
Find out the rate of "false positives" (erroneously detecting disease where none exists) and false negatives (erroneously giving you an all clear when disease does in fact exist) for the tests you have.

➤ You're getting married. Congratulations! You might also be changing health plans (more on this in Chapter 7). If your old plan has better preventive care provisions, you may want to schedule a health assessment before you change. If changing plans requires changing doctors, you may want to have your new doctor do this health assessment.

➤ Are you planning to start a family? Have a check-up first. You may learn about things you can do now to ensure a healthy pregnancy. Find out whether you should enroll your child in your plan or your husband's and what you have to do once the baby is born (more on this in Chapter 7).

133

➤ Adopting? Most adoption agencies require prospective parents to submit evidence of good health. See Chapter 7 about enrolling your adopted child in your plan, and get him or her a comprehensive health assessment.

➤ Sometimes marriage brings a ready-made family. If you are going to cover your stepchildren under your plan, this could be a good time to update their health records with a comprehensive health assessment, especially if they did not have health care coverage before.

➤ Kids have to complete medical forms for school or camp. Use this opportunity to ask any questions you may have about your child's health, behavior, or progress in school. And how about a health assessment for yourself while you're at it?

➤ College students also have to submit medical forms. This is a good opportunity for your child's first comprehensive "grown-up" health assessment.

➤ New job? You may be changing plans or, if it's your first job out of school, getting coverage on your own for the first time. Establishing a relationship with your own doctor is not even as complicated as buying that first post-graduation car, and, we believe, it's more important.

➤ Empty nester? Get a health assessment for yourself *before* turning the kids' bedrooms into photography and art studios.

➤ Your marriage didn't work out. If you're changing health care coverage plans, or changing your status under your ex-spouse's plan, see Chapter 7. If you don't have an up-to-date health assessment, you may want to get one before any plan changes take effect.

Caution

Some jobs require physical examinations. By law, an employer may not require you to undergo such an examination (tests for illegal drug use don't count) unless you have already received a conditional offer of employment. Many managed care plans do not cover employment-related physicals, so ask about cost and who will pay if it's important to you.

➤ Your spouse has died. We're sorry for your loss, and we want you to take care of your health and your coverage. See Chapter 7 or, if you're retired, Chapter 8 and get an updated health assessment, especially if you anticipate changing health care plans.

➤ You've lost your job, or gossip at work says it's possible. Unemployment is physically stressful for many people. It can also lead to gaps in health care coverage. Get a health assessment before your coverage runs out so you can make informed decisions about your coverage and care until you are enrolled in a group plan again.

➤ You're getting ready to retire. You don't need a medical test for that, do you? Well, think again. If you are taking early retirement, you may need to buy your own health care coverage, or get covered under your spouse's plan, until you are eligible for Medicare (which could be decades from now). A health assessment can help you figure out what your best coverage options are and can find medical problems that are best treated before you leave your job. But even if you're retiring at age 65 (and hence eligible for Medicare), a health assessment is a smart idea, especially given the range of coverage options available under Medicare today (covered in Chapter 8).

By now you have the idea. Almost any major change in your life can affect both your health and your health care coverage. A health assessment can help you take the best care of yourself and your family and make the best coverage choices in difficult times.

The Least You Need to Know

➤ If you belong to an HMO, your preventive services are covered. There should be no copays or deductibles, and, if there are, your plan is cheaping out. HMOs' reputations are made on delivering preventive services.

➤ Health screenings and other preventive care are adopted by a plan if they can be applied and be useful to the population as a whole or by age and sex. Your medical history, family history, and risk factors may require more frequent screening.

➤ Forget the annual physical; it's the periodic physical now. You may get your preventive care, then, through cholesterol screenings or height and weight checks. You may also get those height and weight checks, and may catch up on tetanus shots, during a sick visit. The bywords are "Get 'em while you can."

➤ Don't forget that periodic physical. If you're changing plans, it's probably best to see your primary care doctor. And if you're not, there are plenty of milestones to remind you that it's time.

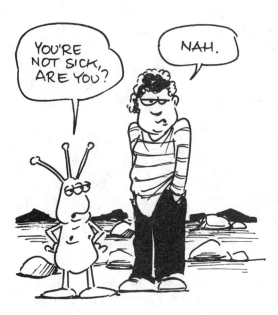

Chapter 13

Men Are from Mars, Women Go to the Doctor

> **In This Chapter**
>
> ➤ How men and women use medical care differently
>
> ➤ A guy's guide to primary care
>
> ➤ Specialty care considerations for men
>
> ➤ Women: deciding between your ob-gyn and internist
>
> ➤ Specialty care considerations for women

It's really true. Men and women use health care differently.

Women spend about 30 years of their lives worrying about getting pregnant (how to, how not to) and its consequences. Women are also still more likely than men to have primary responsibility for their children's medical care (in our experience, this extends to visits to the vet for Fido and Kitty). On a more serious note, women get more cancers at younger ages than men.

Women have more contact with the health care system than men do, in almost all its forms. Women account for 1.5 times as many visits to doctors as men do and 9 percent more visits to hospital emergency rooms. Women also account for 1.5 times as many hospital admissions as men, though their edge narrows to 18 percent when hospitalizations related to pregnancy and delivery are excluded.

Men, on the other hand, are much less likely to get the preventive care they need, in part because they don't face the same biological milestones as women. Men are more likely to enter medical care on their proverbial last leg or bleeding—less predictable occurrences.

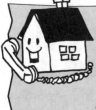

House Call

Though women use the emergency room more, men are 1.25 times as likely as women to go to the emergency room due to an injury. Most fractures among men occur before age 45, while most among women occur at age 65 or older.

Men and women differ not just in body but also in mind. Women are more likely than men to use mental health services, but 2.5 times as many men as women use inpatient and outpatient treatment for alcohol or drug abuse.

Managed care changes not only how we interact with our health plans but also how our health plans expect us to use health care. So, while men and women approach the health care system from different points on the compass—okay, different ends of the universe— we all have to learn how to make the system work to our advantage. This chapter looks at managed care from both the man's and the woman's point of view.

House Call

The five major causes of death in the U.S. are cardiovascular diseases; cancer; accidents and injuries; chronic lung diseases, pneumonia, and influenza; and diabetes mellitus (adult-onset diabetes, often associated with obesity). The most common types of cancer for men involve the prostate, lung, and colon and rectum. The most common types for women involve the breast, colon and rectum, and lung.

Guys: Get Thee to a Doctor

After scouring medical journals and informally surveying friends and relatives, we came to the conclusion that men go to the doctor in large part because they've been hit on the head.

We need to get the guys' attention here, because getting good care under managed care means getting into the system (and knowing how to use it) before stitches, splints, or Code Blue. Guys reading this may say, "You want us to go to the doctor when we're *not sick or bleeding*?" Exactly.

Your father may have touched base with the same doctor once every five or six years when he got sick enough to go. The same doctor may have treated him on that basis for 30 years. You are much more likely than your father to change jobs and health care plans, which may mean changing doctors.

Chapter 11 told you all the reasons getting a primary care doctor in a managed care plan is important. He is your contact, your home base, and your gatekeeper to more care if need be. If you don't bother and the unthinkable happens, you have no one in the system who knows you. Managed care is bureaucratic, and the first rule of dealing with a bureaucracy is to have some allies. If you don't take the time to get a primary care doctor and know how to use him, you are taking pot luck with your life.

One of the ways to do this is to get a periodic health assessment. In an HMO, it's part of your covered services. In a PPO, you may have a specified amount allowed for periodic exams (more on this in Chapter 12). Periodic physical examinations establish what doctors like to call your baseline, or what various parts of your body are supposed to look, feel, and sound like when you're healthy. Changes from this baseline can reflect the ordinary aging process—or something even worse! Having up-to-date medical records may increase your chances of getting appropriate health care when you need it.

House Call

Once upon a time, the annual physical was an important part of many people's medical care. The need for such an annual ritual has largely been debunked, except for people with chronic health conditions or for the elderly, who are prone to more health problems. Many managed care plans, particularly HMOs, cover adult physical examinations, or health assessments, every three years.

That physical also helps you establish a relationship with a primary care doctor who may have to go to bat for you if you need more medical care. And when might that be? When you don't do what you are supposed to do, such as finish your prescription, get refills if your doctor wants you to, or make follow-up appointments.

Here are some easy-to-follow rules for using your primary care doctor:

➤ *Get a primary care doctor when you join your health plan.* Don't just choose the first one on the list; check them out (see Chapter 11 for more on this).

➤ *Know your past.* You are going to have to know your family history, personal health history, and risk factors (smoking, bungee jumping, or both at the same time). Is there a chance that you may have a sexually transmitted disease? Part of what a primary care doctor does is deliver preventive care, and he has to think in terms of screening for certain problems and counseling.

Your Personal Rx
Ask your wife, best friend, or better yet your Mom to help you get ready for a periodic health check-up. Go over your symptoms and family history and write down questions.

➤ *Talk.* Women are used to giving doctors intimate details about their physical state because pregnancy and reproductive health require constant attention. Men don't have that natural segue into the system. You are going to have to give information to the doctor. Write down symptoms and questions. Make the most of your time with him. You don't have to go into the amount of detail you do when you describe the 1985 National League Playoffs, but you do need to relay symptoms.

➤ *Pay attention.* Watch for warning signs and don't downplay the severity of your health problems. If you feel that something is going awry, call the doctor. If your plan has an advice line, call.

Specialty Care for Men: Putting Together a Health Care Team

When you choose your health care plan, you are choosing a team, including specialists if you need them. When you pick a plan, keep in mind the types of specialists you may need to use:

➤ If you are a jock, look at their orthopedists or whether the plan has specialists in sports medicine.

➤ If you suffer from diabetes or high blood pressure, or if heart disease runs in your family, look at the types of specialists in your plan. Check to see if you can go outside the plan for these specialists.

➤ Not old enough to be president yet (35)? This one's for you. The rate of testicular cancer is growing among younger men but has a very high cure rate. Learn how to do monthly exams. Does your plan have the specialists? What are its guidelines for treating testicular cancer?

➤ Skin cancer is more prevalent among men than among women. Again, who are the specialists in your plan? Have you gotten information on identifying skin cancer from your primary care doctor?

➤ Strokes are mankillers. Men are up to ten percent more likely than women to have one, and one out of four men who have strokes will have them before the age of 65. The key to preventing strokes is smoking cessation, keeping blood pressure down, and exercising at least moderately. If you belong to an HMO, it may have programs for all three ready for you to use. If you have any of the risk factors listed above, or a family history of strokes, check with your primary care doctor and make sure your screening is up to date and appropriate for you. Check the caliber of your plan's neurologists and rehabilitation centers, too.

➤ If you are over 40, pay attention to the number and qualifications of urologists on your plan's list. Prostate cancer is the most common cancer in the U.S., second only to lung cancer as a cause of death among men. If you are over 50, check your plan's coverage for second opinions (see Chapter 17). Also check with your plan on its guidelines for testing and treating prostate cancer. This is a complex area, one where being an informed consumer can save your life.

> **Your Personal Rx**
> There is much uncertainty in the diagnosis and treatment of prostate cancer. It's difficult to identify who is at risk of dying of the cancer and those whose disease progresses so slowly that they are more likely to die of something else. If you have a prostate cancer diagnosis, you may want to consider paying out-of-pocket for a second opinion to get an independent diagnosis and treatment recommendation.

Primary and Specialty Care for Women: Who to Choose and When to Use

One of the big debates in managed care today concerns the type of physician who should deliver women's primary care (and sometimes specialty care; more about that below). In some plans, primary care doctors—usually general internists or family practitioners—are expected to carry most of the weight. Other plans, responding in part to pressures from women and their doctors, allow obstetrician/gynecologists (ob-gyns, for short) to serve this function. And some people like nurse practitioners (registered nurses with advanced training in primary care) for their primary care providers, because they often have more time to deal with routine patient concerns.

Who should you choose and when? Following are some of the issues you should think about.

In This Corner, Your Internist

Your internist is supposed to be a Jack or Jill-of-all-trades. He has specialist training in primary care, which means diagnosing and medically treating whatever problems adult patients bring in. Some have a subspecialty, like arthritis or geriatrics. He chose to be an internist because he likes the variety, or perhaps because he likes treating the "whole" person, not just one component. Your internist, however, may not have had gynecological training in med school. You may want to ask about it.

House Call

What is the difference between a family practitioner and an internist? A family practitioner can treat everyone in a family. An internist treats only adults. They both may have some subspecialty or special training to treat a particular age group, such as adolescents or the elderly.

Based on the idealized model of primary care—a place for preventive care, screening, and direction to the next level of care—your primary care doctor should be able to handle your routine gynecological needs. Experts agree that such routine care should include discussions of family planning and prevention of sexually transmitted diseases. Is your doctor willing to deal with these issues and are you comfortable asking? And exactly when does "routine" end and "problem" begin? Will your internist have the experience and detailed understanding to know?

In This Corner, Your Ob-Gyn

Many of a woman's medical needs relate to her reproductive system, whether or not she is sexually active. So an ob-gyn would seem to be a valid choice for primary care. But your ob-gyn trained as a surgeon. Is this the person who will know when that mole should be tested for cancer, or whether you are managing your blood pressure or diabetes correctly?

Many ob-gyn residents are now receiving more training in internal, emergency, and geriatric medicine to make them better able to function as primary care physicians. But that means they will have less training in their own specialty. Some patients may benefit by being able to see a better-rounded ob-gyn as their primary care physician. But what about patients with serious problems who need specialty care?

Many states have direct access laws, allowing you to see your ob-gyn without a referral (see Chapter 11 for more on this). Some HMOs allow you to go to your ob-gyn without a referral when you need routine care.

But don't get a false sense of confidence just because you have direct access to an ob-gyn (that means your primary care doctor doesn't have to okay each visit). If you need treatment for infertility, a problem pregnancy, or a cancer related to your reproductive system, you may need a referral to a subspecialist. You still need a primary care doctor who knows her limits and will argue in your behalf when your treatment needs go beyond her.

It's a Draw

In large part, making this an either-or choice seems a lot like asking, "Do you want pizza or Chinese—forever?" Sure, on Tuesday a large pepperoni with anchovies might hit the spot, but by the weekend our thoughts might turn to moo goo gai pan. We like *both* pizza and Chinese, just on different nights.

If your plan requires you to pick one doctor for your primary care, pick someone competent with whom you can communicate. Can you count on her to work with your plan and your specialists if you need a specialty referral? We're not sure it matters whether this doctor is an internist or ob-gyn, unless you have a chronic condition, such as diabetes, that an ob-gyn would not usually be expected to treat.

If you pick an ob-gyn for a primary doctor, watch for limitations on when you can use one and what she can do. If you can go to your ob-gyn for routine visits without a referral but you need more exams, testing, a referral, or a procedure, you may have to get a referral from your primary care doctor. For instance, if you have a pap smear and it is not within the normal range, you may have to go back to your primary care doctor for a referral to your ob-gyn for further tests. So you will still need a good working relationship with an internist.

Under any circumstances, if your plan allows you an annual visit to your ob-gyn, take advantage of the option. And if you have problems that you fear your doctor(s) is not addressing adequately, ask questions, get second opinions, get referrals (more on this in Chapter 17), or change doctors.

> **Your Personal Rx**
> If your plan requires copayments, your routine ob-gyn may require only your primary care copayment. Other visits may require the specialist copayments. Check your plan handbook and member services to be clear on which copayment may apply to your visit.

House Call

Some managed care plans, particularly those affiliated with university hospitals, are adding women's health centers or contracting with free-standing women's health centers. They are part of the plan and coordinate care, drawing upon the center's specialists in gynecology, obstetrics, endocrinology, internal medicine, cancer, cardiology, psychiatry, and other fields. Best of all, they've added something immensely valuable: extended hours in the mornings and evenings.

Managed Care and Older Women

Managed care changes the way most women over age 50 get medical care. Managed care plans, particularly HMOs, offer valuable screenings for reproductive cancers, osteoporosis, and other conditions important to older women. Women over 50 also have more illnesses and use more prescriptions than men, and spend more on prescription drugs.

The Older Women's League, an advocacy group, suggests women over 50 ask the following questions when choosing a managed care plan:

➤ Ask about coverage limitations, preapproval requirements for specialists, whether you can get care out of the network, and, if so, how much the plan pays for that care.

➤ Find out what specialists a plan has in its network and what you should do if you cannot see a specialist promptly.

➤ Ask about prescription benefits and how to get drugs not on the plan's formulary list (see also Chapter 16).

➤ Learn about grievance procedures (see Chapter 23 for more on this).

Much of medicine is playing catch-up on how to deliver the right health care to women overall. In the past, women were routinely excluded from federally financed clinical studies because of concerns about pregnancy, birth defects, and menstrual and hormonal fluctuations, and how these situations could affect both the patient's health and the validity of research results. Consequently, most drug trials for drugs important to women as they age—such as those for treating heart ailments, arthritis, and high blood pressure—were tested on men.

House Call

In 1990, the U.S. National Institutes of Health created an office to set a research agenda for women's health and track the inclusion of women in clinical trials. The year 2006 will bring the conclusion of a 15-year study of women ages 50 to 79 through the Women's Health Initiative. The study focuses on heart disease, cancer, and osteoporosis, and covers lifestyles, attitude, diet, and medications.

Doctors for Men and Women: At Your Side and on Your Side

The potential high impact of many plan exclusions on women's health makes it especially important for women to consult doctors with experience in managed care—and the will to persevere—as well as significant experience in the problem being treated. It may not be enough to deal with a doctor you trust and are comfortable with if the doctor does not also have the experience and expertise to justify his or her decisions to your plan. Here are some examples:

➤ If a plan excludes experimental procedures, your doctor should know never to use the terms "experimental" or "investigational" in justifying your treatment (most experts in advanced procedures will know this).

➤ If you have a medical need for surgery that will have cosmetic improvement as a side benefit and your plan excludes cosmetic surgery, your doctor should ignore any cosmetic improvements in requesting authorization from your plan.

Will Your Doctor Fight the Good Fight?

Your doctor's personality can also make a difference in negotiating managed care plans on your behalf. In some of the better managed care plans, a clerk or a nurse can approve a treatment plan that calls for preauthorization, but only another doctor—often right there in the same office as a clerk or a nurse—can *deny* a doctor's treatment request or specialist referral. In plans that don't follow this procedure, your doctor may need to ask to talk to someone's supervisor or, preferably, to a physician.

Will your doctor take the time to learn your plan's bureaucracy? It's a part of modern patient care, but some doctors see the need for such follow-up as an intrusion. And will your doctor risk being dropped from the plan if that's the price of fighting for your best care?

Stay Up to Date

Good specialist care is especially important in areas of medicine where knowledge about diagnosis and treatment is changing rapidly. You don't want to be the last person in the country to have an unnecessary mastectomy or prostatectomy, do you? Be wary of doctors who tell you that you have only one treatment choice (with cancer, for example, this is often not the case). What you are hearing could reflect the plan's philosophy—or fee schedule—rather than evolving medical practice. If you are uneasy, ask to change doctors or get a second opinion.

Have It Your Way

Most good doctors will want you to take an active part in your treatment decisions, especially if you are facing a serious medical problem. We, too, favor equality in the doctor-patient relationship and urge you to explore all your treatment options.

But this may not be your style. If you are facing a serious medical problem, you may prefer to have the doctor make your decisions. If that is the case, many experts believe you should just *tell her*. You're facing enough stress without having to conform to some-one else's view of the model patient (even ours!). Your relationship with your doctor will be much improved if you both know what to expect from each other. But you still have to keep tabs on what your plan requires you to do in the course of your treatment; your doctor's office may let something fall through the cracks.

House Call

Areas of medicine where knowledge is changing rapidly can pose special challenges to the informed consumer. Excellent popular guides are now available for many conditions. However, by the time a book on a fast-changing topic is published, parts can be out of date. Read all you can, then tell your doctor what you have read and ask him to update you.

The Least You Need to Know

➤ Men and women use medical care differently. But there are rules that apply to both: Pick a good primary care doctor and take advantage of age- and gender-specific health screenings.

➤ When you choose a plan, look at the specialist roster for an indication of how well your plan can treat gender-specific diseases.

➤ Men, make sure you get a primary care doctor as soon as you join a plan. Don't wait until you need stitches or open-heart surgery.

➤ Women, make sure you know how and when you can use your ob-gyn. Sometimes you can go without a referral, but sometimes that freedom applies only to routine visits. If your plan allows her to be your primary care doctor, think about how you would use her and whether she fits the bill for your main doctor.

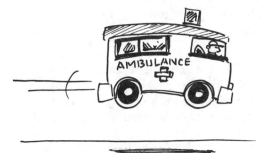

Emergency Care: Smart Moves and Common Sense

It's 2 a.m., and the baby's fever hits 104°. Or your hands swell and your throat tightens a half hour after you take an antibiotic. You know you're supposed to follow a special drill for emergency care, but you don't know exactly what to do first or where to find instructions.

How fast and clearly can you think during an emergency? Sometimes you will be the person making the decision about whether to seek emergency care; sometimes you will be the patient helping someone else make the right decision for you. This chapter will help you make the right choices during the difficult, confusing, and painful times that happen to all of us.

Prepare in Advance—Because You Never Know

In every contact with managed care, preparation is key. You are dealing with a business that depends on procedures, permissions, and reviews. These rules are not necessarily complicated, but you need to know and use them.

When you sign up with your health plan, read the materials your plan sends you, such as plan documents and handbooks, and see what to do in an emergency. Make sure you do this before anything happens. Most often, the rules for emergency care will be in a separate section in your member handbook. It explains what is an emergency or urgent and lists examples of each. If your state uses the *prudent layperson standard*, your handbook probably mentions it.

Healthspeak
Under the *prudent layperson standard*, emergency care is covered if the decision to go to the ER was one that an average person with average medical knowledge would make at the time.

If you have questions, ask your primary care doctor right away or ask the plan's member services department. Add a bookmark to (sticky notes are great) the emergency care section in your member handbook and circle or highlight it. You may need to react quickly, so make it easy for yourself.

If your employer holds meetings during health plan enrollment season, ask the managed care plan representatives about emergency care, whether they use the prudent layperson or another standard, and which hospitals they use. If you have children, ask about access to pediatric emergency care.

House Call
Talk to your primary care physician or pediatrician about how to handle emergencies or urgent care under your plan. He may have suggestions on recognizing and handling emergency and urgent situations, and on which hospitals to use.

Make sure your baby-sitters, caretakers, and family members also know what to do. Leave a simple set of written instructions and telephone numbers. If you've programmed 911 on your telephone, also program your advice and urgent care line numbers. Some plans may be understanding if your baby-sitter or grandma dashes to the ER without following your plan's rules, but there is no guarantee.

The rules for emergency care may be the same even if you are out of town. Your member handbook should have a section on what is called "out-of-service area" care. You may still have to call the advice or urgent care line if you are not sure it is an emergency, and they will instruct you how to proceed.

Also check if in fact you will be covered for out-of service area emergency care. Managing your care includes putting the stops on circumstances where you are likely to incur emergency expenses outside the plan, and your handbook or contract will list those circumstances. Sometimes care is not covered if the patient "could have reasonably foreseen the necessity for care prior to leaving the service area," so if you have a fever, sore neck, and severe sore throat before leaving town, check in with your primary care doctor.

Your handbook also will explain how to notify the plan if you are hospitalized. Make sure that someone checks (or knows to check) with the plan to see if the hospital has done so. If you use a hospital that participates in your plan, the hospital may be required to notify the plan and take care of preauthorizations for you.

> **Your Personal Rx**
> Special warning to women who are seven or more months pregnant, terminally ill people, or people with unstable conditions: You may need prior approval from the plan's medical director before leaving town. Otherwise, the plan may not cover even emergency care you need while away.

Is It Urgent, an Emergency, or Can It Wait Until Monday?

The managed care mantra for *emergency* care is that the emergency room is for serious injuries or life-threatening medical conditions. These are the here and now, life-threatening or maiming events that *must* be conquered.

An *emergency* is a sudden, unexpected onset of a condition or an injury that requires immediate medical or surgical care. Delay could endanger life or cause permanent disability. An *urgent* condition needs treatment within 24 hours to prevent it from turning into a serious or life-threatening illness. It could be treated by your primary care doctor or, if available, an urgent care clinic.

The plan doesn't want you using the ER for an earache, a cold, or a long-standing back problem. There are several reasons for this:

> **Healthspeak**
> An *emergency* is the sudden onset of a condition or an injury requiring immediate medical or surgical care. An *urgent* condition, in contrast, needs treatment within 24 hours to prevent it from turning into a serious or life-threatening illness. An urgent care clinic provides care for problems that need to be treated outside routine business hours but that are not serious enough to require emergency room care.

➤ ER care is more costly than the same care delivered in another setting, such as a doctor's office.

➤ The ER is the place where, unlike Cheers, the famous TV bar, *nobody* knows your name. They also don't know your health status, medical records, or medical history. You get better health care if the doctor treating you knows something about you. In a true emergency, of course, this doesn't matter as much as saving your life.

➤ "If it bleeds, it leads." No matter how uncomfortable you are, you may be waiting for hours as people with gunshot wounds, auto accident injuries, and heart attacks are treated.

"Emergency" *does not* mean "fast service" unless *the ER staff*, not you, think your case is serious. And even severe inconvenience to you does not necessarily make for an emergency. Your child's earache may keep you up all night, but that doesn't make it an emergency.

Here is where your goal and the plan's may differ. You want to know what the problem is and get it fixed. The plan wants to decide whether your case is serious enough to stabilize at the ER, or can it be fixed elsewhere?

Feeling vulnerable? Afraid you'll make the wrong move? You are not alone. Even ER personnel tell us that the answers are often not black and white. Extremely serious problems may be present without affecting every *vital sign* (temperature, pulse, blood pressure, and respiration). On the other hand, what is very painful and seems serious may be treated just as well, or better, in your doctor's office or an *urgent care* clinic.

Healthspeak
Vital signs are the patient's temperature, pulse, blood pressure, and respiration. A first-aid course or good first-aid book will tell you how to measure and evaluate these signs.

Some managed care plans cover ER care only if it turns out to actually have been an emergency, not if you believed it was an emergency at the time. But the trend, and in some states the law, is a prudent layperson standard.

Under the prudent layperson standard, a decision to go to the ER is covered if it is one that an average person with average medical knowledge would make *at the time*. Medicare, the health care component of Social Security, uses this standard.

Your Personal Rx
Some managed care companies may not take calls on a 24-hour basis for precertifications, that is, an advance review of the need for hospital admission. If your plan's precertification line is closed, make sure someone makes the calls on the next working day.

If you *do* go to the ER, don't be surprised if you are moved quickly. You will be moved after you are stabilized. Many managed care plans contract with businesses that assess whether a patient is stable and then moves him or her to a hospital with which they contract for services. This process keeps their costs down. These assessment firms even bring the ambulance and ride to the hospital with you.

The following sections discuss the steps to take when you suspect an emergency.

Call

If it's obviously an emergency—someone has lost consciousness, for example—call 911 (or another emergency number if your area doesn't use 911). Check with your primary care doctor, advice line, or urgent care line if you are less certain. For example, a high fever in a child is usually not an emergency unless the child is displaying other symptoms such as listlessness or inconsolable crying.

There is usually a separate number to call if your plan steers you to urgent care lines. The advice and urgent care numbers will be in your plan materials, the plan's newsletter (if it publishes one), and possibly on your membership card. Urgent care lines are typically staffed by registered nurses. They are either part of your plan or in business to service managed care plans. They'll make the call on your care based on plan experience and guidelines for responding to urgent and emergency calls. Yes, it is another card in your wallet, but the card lists the phone number to call and steps to take in dealing with emergencies. If you do not follow this procedure, the financial burden may be shifted to you.

Remember: You never give up your right to call an emergency number because you belong to a managed care plan. You are not precluded from getting to the hospital on time. The consequences of going to the ER even though your plan says no or later decides it was not necessary are financial alone. Financial consequences can be substantial, but risking permanent harm or even death to you or your family is worse.

Tell All

After conducting an unscientific survey of the human race, we believe there are two types of humans: those who fall apart during an emergency, and those who fall apart afterward. We all need a little help to be the best we can be during stressful times.

When you call, give all the information you can about the patient's condition, but don't waste time giving a diagnosis. You weren't trained as an ER doctor. That's *their* job. Your best weapon is your ability to describe the problem. Be as precise as you can:

➤ Describe the ABCs first—airways, breathing, and circulation: If any airways are blocked (for instance, choking on food) whether the person has labored, shallow or has no breathing and has a part of the body gone numb or is the person turning blue.

➤ Symptoms: where it hurts, how often, and what the patient's temperature is.

➤ Chronology: when the symptoms started, when they got worse, or when the accident occurred.

➤ Vital extras: patient's age; medications he or she is taking; chronic illnesses such as asthma, diabetes, and so on; and special circumstances, such as where, when, and what the patient ate.

Focus on describing what you see, feel, and remember. Many plans hand out, or make available at a discount, easy-to-use books about illnesses and emergency situations with descriptions of symptoms. Use the words in the book. For instance, if the book says "a cough that sounds like a seal," and your child does sound like a seal, you know your description is familiar to the person on the other end of the line. If you say, "It sounds like when my Aunt Mannie had TB," that may not ring a bell with the urgent care nurse.

It's Your Call

Caution

An "urgent" situation can turn into an "emergency." For instance, severe abdominal pain may require urgent care. But if it becomes continuous, accompanied by vomiting, it may indicate a life-threatening illness. Keep in contact with your primary care doctor or the advice line during the whole episode.

Your Personal Rx

If you leave the ER with a prescription and can wait to fill it on the way home, you may be able to save some money. Some hospital pharmacies aren't part of the managed care plan, so it may be better to go to a pharmacy that is.

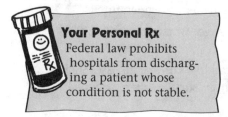

Your Personal Rx

Federal law prohibits hospitals from discharging a patient whose condition is not stable.

Step three is your decision: Is it an emergency, urgent, or should you wait for an appointment? If you and your doctor or urgent care contact decide that it is not a true emergency but requires immediate care, you have several options. Get in to see your doctor. If it is after hours or on the weekend, some plans have their own contracts with urgent care centers. And home visits are actually making a comeback in some areas, especially for pediatricians. It often saves money for the plan and saves the pediatrician on call the distress of making the wrong decision.

Follow Up

Step four is to keep in touch and be persistent. If you get worse despite the advice of your doctor or plan, let them know. If you go to the ER, tell them what you've done and that you have gotten worse despite taking their advice. There are many stories about people who were released from the ER or urgent care facility, went back, were released again, and then became critically ill or died. If you follow up, you reduce the chances that this will happen to you.

If you go to the ER, a screening exam should be done. If you get worse and go back a second time to no avail, ask to see another doctor. Ask about staying on for a limited time for observation. Be warned, however, that you take a chance that your plan may not be willing to pay if your situation does not turn out to be an emergency.

Stay in touch with your own physician and get her to the hospital if necessary. Managed care plans place a premium on contact, continuity, and control. You should do the same. Make sure you get instructions for follow-up care and make arrangements right after you leave the ER. If you keep up the contact and continuity, it enhances your own ability to maintain control.

Psychiatric Emergencies

What do you do in a psychiatric emergency? What if it can't wait overnight? According to the American College of Emergency Physicians, suicidal or homicidal feelings are considered warning signs of emergencies.

Sometimes your plan will have separate telephone numbers for mental health and substance abuse services. You will most likely be required to obtain precertification for hospitalization for psychiatric or substance abuse just as for any other admission. Ask your plan what to do in case of emergency and what numbers to call (more on this in Chapter 19).

The managed care plan will want to transfer you to one of its facilities or treatment centers. Managed care emphasizes keeping costs down, and outpatient care is cheaper than inpatient care. For instance, if you want to be admitted for chemical dependency and haven't failed in outpatient care, the plan will push for outpatient care first. This rule may be waived in a true psychiatric or medical emergency.

> **Caution**
> Adults must go through a legal process before being involuntarily admitted for psychiatric care. In most states, the parent or guardian makes that decision for a child and usually must be present to consent to admission.

Sometimes you will get conflicting signals from the hospital staff and the managed care plan. After all, the hospital staff is right there, while the managed care plan representative may be on the other end of a telephone line. (Their goals may also be different: To the hospital you are a paying customer, while to the plan you are a cost item.) Managed care plans often have an "assessor" on site before you are even seen in the ER to make sure you are an appropriate candidate for admission.

The person must not be a threat to his or her own safety or the safety of others before they can be released. However, it is up to the managed care plan, patient, and family (if involved or the patient is a minor) for the next steps in treatment.

Special Cases: Kids and the Elderly

Emergencies involving children and the elderly can be particularly vexing. Emergencies may vary by age. Children and the elderly can present different symptoms for critical conditions such as shock. Kids and seniors may also not be able to explain things clearly—or even at all.

These factors may make it more difficult for you to distinguish between emergencies and urgent situations. That's why giving as precise a description as you can to the urgent care line or physician can sometimes be a lifesaver.

When a Child Is Sick

Managed care plans are very aware that parents have relied on the emergency room far more than necessary. Most children get better, even with high fevers, and much of pediatric medicine is better delivered by the family pediatrician than in the ER. You've probably read or heard stories about urgent care lines giving the wrong information, or waiting too long before approving a trip to the hospital. Once again, your best resource is knowing what to do before an emergency strikes and your ability to describe what is happening.

> **Your Personal Rx**
> After vital signs, airway, and breathing, the best indicators of emergency in a child is the child's behavior. Is she inconsolable? Is he lethargic, unable to be aroused? Has there been an injury or other trauma? What's his temperature? These are the parameters the doctors will use.

> **Your Personal Rx**
> If an allergy is life-threatening, get your child a bracelet or necklace with the allergy information on it. Make sure your child's school health form is up to date, and put a copy of key medical data in a zipper pocket of your child's backpack.

Before you join a plan, ask where children are taken in case of emergency and find out if they have pediatric emergency departments. It may make a difference in the type of plan you choose. Also, ask your pediatrician what hospital she prefers for emergency services, and see if your plan covers that preference. Her experience is invaluable.

Don't minimize the importance of calling the urgent care line, unless it is obviously an emergency. If you don't check in, the likelihood is that even coverage based on a prudent layperson assessment of emergency may be denied. Many ER doctors told us that parents often ran directly to the emergency room out of panic, confusion, or frustration. High fevers or symptoms of ear infections can bring on a parental panic attack. All of the above responses are part of being a parent. Take a deep breath, keep your wits, and recognize that, with some help, you most likely will make the right decision.

If your child is under treatment for a chronic condition or on medication, tell the urgent care line and, if you go, the emergency room. Often, parents don't have information on their child's specialist or medication. Keep your pediatrician's card in your wallet, and write the name and telephone number of the specialist on the back, along with the medication and dosage. Having only one card to deal with may make it easier for you to respond quickly to questions. Keeping your child's physicians in the loop will also give you something important to your child and to the managed care plan—continuity of care.

The Elderly

Elderly people may pose other problems in a crisis. They may have distorted perceptions of pain (not feeling it or feeling slight pain excessively) and time (not being able to tell you how long a symptom has persisted). So if you are caring for an elderly person, you may have to be more cautious in deciding whether to go to the ER.

As always, the patient's personal profile substantially affects emergency decisions, but especially in the case of the elderly who may have accumulated a long list of chronic conditions. Relate important information such as age, condition or health status, family history, temperature, and medications immediately to the urgent care line. If you go or are taken to the emergency room, try to relay medications, prior episodes, and names of physicians as soon as you can, or have someone do it for you.

House Call

Five symptoms that may signal a medical emergency in the elderly are confusion; lethargy or feeling of weakness; low-grade fever; labored or rapid breathing; and mild abdominal discomfort.

If your visit to the emergency room is reviewed by Medicare or by your supplemental plan, make sure the reviewer knows about statements you may have made to family and friends during the episode, such as, "I think I'm having a heart attack." They can be used during a review of the layperson's assessment of the risk of permanent damage.

Your Common Sense Is Your Best Guide

One thing has not changed in the move to managed care: Your common sense is your best friend in an emergency. When we talked to ER and primary care doctors and nurses, we were told over and over that you should "listen to your gut."

In a true emergency, your plan will pay for treatment at the closest facility. If you are admitted to a hospital, assume you must notify your plan within 24 hours. Find out if the hospital has done so. Follow up on it yourself or let someone know they should follow up for you. The plan's objective is to start using physicians and hospitals under contract as soon as possible, so notification is very important.

Your Personal Rx

Your plan may refuse to pay for ER services if you don't provide adequate information supporting the ER visit. Answer all information requests from the plan that you receive after the visit. Your chances of the plan paying will be much improved.

What if your plan thinks you've made a mistake, and it was not an emergency? Appeal. Get copies of intake documents and records. If other people were with you when you were injured or became sick, get their statements. If you prevail, you don't have to pay. If you've followed the rules of the plan and maintained contact and continuity, you have a better chance of prevailing.

What (and Whom) to Take with You to the ER

If you head to the emergency room, there may be no time to prepare, so have a simple plan in place at all times:

➤ Keep your plan I.D. card with you. Have your kids carry their cards or plan information with them as soon as they are old enough to carry a wallet, and definitely by the time they carry a driver's license.

➤ Keep your emergency numbers (including your urgent care number) at hand or programmed on your phone. If you are taking medication, tell someone to bring it to the ER with you.

➤ Make sure you know what your plan asks you to do in case of emergency. Fill out copies of the Life Saver form (on the following page) for each member of the family, and keep it where you or someone else can find it fast. If at all possible, grab your member handbook.

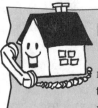

House Call

Emergency medical technicians and paramedics—the people who respond to 911 calls—say that if you have an allergy or a severe condition, wear a bracelet or necklace. During an emergency call, they don't rifle through your purse or pockets for information for fear of being accused of theft.

➤ If at all possible, take someone who can act as an advocate for you when you can't act as one for yourself. There are two reasons this is important: You need that extra dose of common sense in order to answer the ER's questions clearly, and it's useful to have someone who can attest to your reasons for going to the emergency room if that ever becomes a question.

Your Life Saver
Medical Contact and Information Form

Date_____

Name_____ DOB_____ / _____ / _____

Work Phone_____ Home Phone_____

Work Address_____
Home Address_____

_____

_____

Primary Care Doctor or Pediatrician
Name_____ Phone No._____

Specialist (If Applicable)
Name_____ Phone No._____

Current Medications

_____

_____

Major Medical Problems or Chronic Conditions

_____

_____

Allergies _____

Date of Last Tetanus Booster_____ Blood Type_____

IN CASE OF EMERGENCY, PLEASE CALL
(Parent/Guardian of Minor, Next of Kin)
Name/Relationship/Phone No. _____ **Cell/Pager** _____

Name/Relationship/Phone No. _____

Name/Relationship/Phone No. _____

MY HEALTH CARE COMPANY INFORMATION

Name of Health Care Plan _____

Phone _____

Utilization Review Dept. _____

ID No. _____ Plan No. _____

Organ Donor?   Yes _____   No _____   Health Care Proxy?   Yes _____   No _____

Living Will?   Yes _____   No _____

The Least You Need to Know

➤ Emergency means serious injury or the onset of life-threatening medical problems. It does not mean inconvenience—even severe pain and other discomfort.

➤ "Urgent" and "emergency" aren't the same thing. But what starts out urgent may turn into an emergency, so keep in contact with your primary care physician and/or urgent care line after your first call.

➤ Be sure you understand what you are required to do when you have a serious situation. Also make sure that any baby-sitters, relatives, or caretakers have easy-to-follow instructions in an emergency.

➤ Keep those health care cards in your wallet. Know the numbers to call and the hospitals that serve you.

➤ In a true medical emergency, go to the nearest hospital or dial 911, then call or make sure someone else calls the health plan.

➤ If it is not a clear medical emergency, be sure to call your health plan first as instructed in your member handbook.

➤ If you are far along in pregnancy (35 plus weeks) or seriously or terminally ill, check with your plan's medical director before leaving town. It may affect how you get medical care outside the service area and if your plan will pay for it.

Part 4
Above and Beyond: When You Need Special Care

Need help with your health? You can bet that at some time you or a loved one will need special care for health problems that are out of the ordinary. Can (and will) your plan meet your needs? What can you do to make sure your plan is on top of the latest treatments?

Almost everyone at some time crosses out of primary care territory and into the land of a medical specialist. This is someone who specializes in just one part or area of the body (or soul). You may want to consult a specialist about having a baby, treating a chronic condition or major illness, finding out about the newest treatments for what ails you, or conquering mental health or substance abuse problems.

Special circumstances can also arise if you need medical care while out of town or if you want something different from what standard medicine offers you. We're also sure you will agree that the "little extras" many plans offer to keep you healthy and happy are pretty special, too.

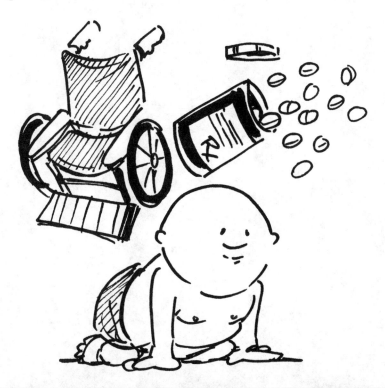

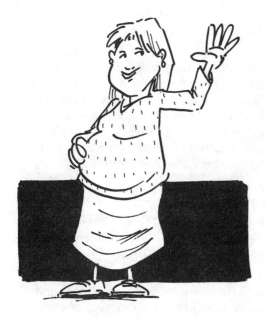

Chapter 15

Maternity Care: Nine Months and Counting

In This Chapter

➤ Planning ahead for your trip to parenthood

➤ Choosing your obstetrician: a critical choice

➤ Next on your itinerary—prenatal visits

➤ At-risk pregnancies

➤ Reaching your destination: delivery and after

If you are pregnant, an exciting journey is about to begin. You will be poked and prodded. You will talk about your family, siblings, parents, and grandparents more than at your last reunion. You will lose sight of your toes. *And* you will be more closely involved with the medical system, and your managed care plan, than at any other time in your life. This chapter gives you the information you need to get good maternity care.

Planning Ahead

If you are planning to get pregnant, put maternity care high on the list of things to consider when picking a plan. Obstetric care is often part of plan report cards and quality reports (see Chapter 6 for more on this). How many mothers received prenatal care in the first trimester? What is the percentage of pregnancies resulting in Cesareans (C-sections)? What is the number of women who had normal delivery after having had a C-section for a previous delivery? These facts will make a lot of difference to you during those nine months.

Take a good look at how "deep" the plan is. Does it have enough obstetricians for its members? Does it have obstetric specialists? There are some days when more babies are delivered than others (what is it with snowstorms?), but you want a plan that doesn't consistently overburden its obstetricians.

You may also want to check out if the plan pays for family planning. If you are having difficulty conceiving or carrying a child to term, check out if your plan covers infertility services, the scope of those services, where they are delivered, and how much the plan pays.

Be prepared. And be prepared to be vigilant. This journey can have many twists and turns. Panic gives way to optimism, and confidence gives way to uncertainty. After talking to many mothers, and from personal experiences, it seems that the best—and the worst—of a health plan comes to the surface during these nine months.

Your Personal Rx
A word of motherly advice from someone who has been there. Get a pedicure. When your toes finally reappear, you don't want them in any way to resemble what you've just gone through.

Your Personal Rx
Watch for changes to your benefits during your pregnancy. And continue to check on your maternity benefits. Health plans often change some of the benefits they offer when a new plan year begins. Pay attention to any communications from your plan.

Choosing an Obstetrician

And the nomination for the person who, during labor, you swear you will never see again is…your obstetrician!

We've heard that some have nominated their husbands, but, after all the trips to your obstetrician's office and all the tests, questions, and discomfort in the examining room, you will need a break from her, too.

Those intense feelings come from the experience of an intimate involvement with your obstetrician. You're trusting her with the lives of yourself and your child. You have to have a sense of security, which means you have to be confident in her abilities and assured of open, two-way communication.

Check out your plan's list. Use some of the same criteria listed for your primary care doctor, such as certification, training, specialties, and location (after driving a stick shift home from the obstetrician's office during early labor, one of the authors can attest to the value of location). Other questions include:

➤ How long have you practiced in this type of managed care setting?

➤ What is your philosophy of care?

➤ What arrangements do you have if complications occur? (It's very important to be satisfied with this answer.)

➤ Who can be present during labor and birth?

If you've chosen a gynecologist for your gynecological exams or, if your plan allows, as your primary care doctor, you may want to continue with the same person for obstetrical care. But be sure and check her out. If you have the potential of a problem or at-risk pregnancy and your gynecologist does not have much experience, ask for her recommendation. If you've met your gynecologist only for your exam and spent a total of two hours over the past four years with her, check her out the same way you would any new obstetrician.

And don't forget one of the best resources—other mothers. Information from personal experience about both the obstetricians and the plan can be invaluable.

Can Your Choice Include a Nurse-Midwife?

The use of *certified nurse-midwives* is a changing picture. Sometimes they can provide maternity care only, and sometimes they can deliver the full scope of maternity, family planning, preconception care, newborn care, and preventive services. Often, it is difficult to tell from the plan's directory if nurse-midwives are included. If they are used in conjunction with an obstetric practice, as in a PPO or an IPA, they may not be listed separately in your provider directory.

If you want a nurse-midwife to see you through your pregnancy, ask the following:

➤ Are nurse-midwives included in the plan?

Caution

Not every gynecologist (specialist in women's health) is also board-certified in obstetrics (the branch of medicine concerned with the treatment of women during pregnancy, childbirth, and immediately following). In fact, some gynecologists may avoid obstetrical practice to reduce their medical liability insurance costs. Make sure your doctor is qualified and willing to treat you.

Healthspeak

A *certified nurse-midwife* is a health-care practitioner educated in the two disciplines of nursing and midwifery. That person has graduated from an accredited school of midwifery, acquired national certification, and is licensed to practice in the state. To check on certification, you can call the Association of Certified Nurse Midwives Certification Council, Inc., at (301)459-1321. Their Website is at **http://acnmcertcn @aol.com.**

➤ In what settings will the plan pay for nurse-midwife services? Remember, nurse midwives usually don't deliver high-risk births.

➤ Does the plan cover births in a freestanding birth center (a choice that is being offered more frequently by managed care plans)?

Then ask the nurse-midwife the same questions about credentials, training, and experience that you would ask a doctor.

Can You Afford to See a Practitioner Not in Your Plan?

Get out your pencil, paper, and calculator, because babies can cost a bundle. One of the strengths of HMOs is their full coverage of prenatal care. But if you don't like what you see (or experience) and want to go elsewhere, those many visits and hospital care can add up in the thousands. Even if your HMO has a point-of-service plan, the cost of frequent visits can't be ignored.

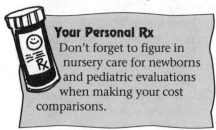

Your Personal Rx
Don't forget to figure in nursery care for newborns and pediatric evaluations when making your cost comparisons.

Make sure to get the facts and figures from your health plan from the beginning. Should you trade the $10 copayment per visit for an out-of-pocket expense of over $100 each time? If you have a POS, how much is the copayment? What percentage of the delivery does the plan pay? If you don't use your PPO list, what percentage of prenatal care and hospital care does the plan pay? If you want to use a nurse-midwife, will the plan pay for it?

Double check those figures with your plan. This is not the time for surprises, and a "surprise" can run into the thousands of dollars. For example, a baby born prematurely or with problems can run up hundreds of thousands of dollars in the neonatal intensive care unit.

If, after all these considerations, you want to go to someone outside your plan, you may save money by asking both her and your plan if they want each other. PPOs and IPAs may be on the lookout for doctors who are referred by members, and doctors may take a second look at a plan if patients are asking them to join.

Prenatal Visits

Let's take one step back. It may be a good idea to have a prepregnancy exam. Racial and ethnic groups with inherited diseases, such as sickle cell anemia and Tay-Sachs disease, may want testing to determine whether the baby is likely to have the disease. An exam is also helpful if you have a preexisting illness such as diabetes or epilepsy. Sexually transmitted diseases and rubella exposure that may harm the baby can also be identified at this time.

For the good health of both you and your baby, start prenatal care early; it pays off for everyone. Most health care plans pay for prenatal visits, though some require a copayment. Make that visit as soon as your pregnancy is confirmed. If you are choosing an obstetrician for the first time, or a new one, be sure to allot enough time. The first visit is usually time intensive.

The first visit should occur no later than 12 weeks after conception. It usually includes:

➤ A medical history

➤ Physical examination (including pelvic)

➤ Laboratory tests

Your medical history is extremely important here, so find someone with whom you feel free to talk. You have to inform them about medications you take, including antidepressants, previous or chronic health conditions, family history, including genetic-related conditions such as Huntington's disease, cystic fibrosis, or mental retardation. Also discuss drugs and alcohol use (see Chapter 22 for information on medical records and confidentiality) as well as previous pregnancies, including abortions and miscarriages.

Your visits may then keep a particular schedule, or you may require more attention. Be sure you schedule according to the doctor's request at the time you leave the office.

Between 15 and 20 weeks into the pregnancy, you will receive two important tests: an ultrasound and a blood screening called a maternal serum alpha-fetoprotein test (MSAFP). These are important and need to be done at specific times. A good ultrasound is very important. It can find structural birth defects, heart and kidney problems, minor defects such as cleft palates, determine the number of fetuses (you want to know, don't you?), and help set the due date. An MSAFP screening can detect some neural tube defects (those of the spine and brain) and help identify women whose babies are at risk for certain other abnormalities like Down's syndrome.

A high or low test doesn't necessarily indicate the baby has an abnormality. It may mean other things, such as twins or vaginal bleeding. It is an indication to look further. Make sure you understand the information your are given. If further tests are required, find out what steps you should take to get the tests done at the right time.

Your other visits will include size and weight measurements, and checks on the baby's position. Another special testing occurs at 24 weeks when a glucose tolerance test is administered to make sure you don't have diabetes brought on by the pregnancy.

One of the best questions to ask at almost any stage of pregnancy, whether it is carefree or wrought with complications, is "Why is the treatment you recommended the best treatment for me?" Make sure you keep a record of the answers from both the doctor and the plan.

Your Personal Rx

Pregnancy-related programs may be available through your plan. Many HMOs offer childbirth classes through the plan, and others offer postpartum "coping" classes, as well as early childhood classes for no or nominal cost.

Life in the High-Tech Lane

If your prenatal blood tests show that there may be a problem, or you are over age 35, your doctor may recommend one of two tests: chorionic villus sampling (CVS) or amniocentisis. CVS is done at 10 to 13 weeks, and amniocentisis is done at around 14 weeks. These tests can give a wealth of information about the baby.

House Call

Older mothers, who have a higher risk of giving birth to a Down's syndrome baby, and families with a history of sickle cell anemia should consult the March of Dimes for excellent information about prenatal tests and what they can (and cannot) show.

If you do have a family history of genetic disorders, now is a good time to ask your obstetrician about genetic tests that may be available during your pregnancy. You also have to ask yourself what you will do with that information. Genetic counselors told us that if you are clear about your approach to what you may hear with your obstetrician, you'll have a better working relationship with her about the tests and the results.

As with any testing, make sure to ask what the risks and benefits are of having the test done.

If you require further testing, now is the time to keep tabs on your physician and your plan. Sometimes referrals may be required for these tests, so keep tabs on whether they should come from your obstetrician or primary care doctor. If very specialized testing is suggested, you may need an out-of-network referral. If a fetal abnormality emerges, it may also require repeated referrals.

These can be difficult situations. Sometimes the genetic counselors at the hospital labs where the initial testing is done are good at explaining the pregnancy screening and test results to whichever doctor is empowered to give referrals. It is wise to put on your "advocate" hat, arm yourself with information, and carefully weigh what your plan, doctor, and you want to do.

High-Risk Pregnancies

Pregnancies are considered high-risk when a woman has certain medical conditions that automatically place a woman in the high-risk category. These may include a pregnant woman older than age 35 or one with diabetes, heart or lung disease, high blood pressure, sexually transmitted disease, or thyroid or neurological problems. Make sure you have copies of any reports used to evaluate whether yours is a high-risk pregnancy so that you can use them to evaluate your care.

If you are in that category, or think you may be at some point in your pregnancy, check out the plan and see if the specialists they tout are truly specialists. It's not enough to have delivered at-risk moms. Do they have any special training? The question to ask is "Have you had experience and training delivering women like me, not just women in the high-risk category?"

This is the time to learn the referral process cold. If you are stonewalled, you may have to act fast. You may have to muster support—medical, legal, and financial—to get what you want. (For more on specialists, referrals, and what to do when you disagree with the plan, see Chapters 16, 17, and 23.)

Time is of the essence. Though some chronic conditions can be managed by primary care doctors, pregnancies can complicate a condition like insulin-dependent diabetes and should be handled by specialists.

Check your plan to see what treatments, medications, or hospitalizations may not be covered. If you have any questions, make sure you ask member services and make sure your doctor knows if there are limitations. If your doctor is on the list for 20 plans, it may be difficult for her to keep 20 specific plan restrictions in mind.

> **Your Personal Rx**
> If you have a chronic disease and your plan limits you to the primary care doctor for prenatal and maternity care, use your regular specialist to get information you need about your condition as it relates to your pregnancy.

Delivery and After

Somewhere after the seventh month, you will fill out preadmission forms. Be sure to bring your health plan card. Now, a preadmission requirement may sound odd, after all these months of doctor's visits, tests, and preparation. But if your plan requires preadmission and you don't do it, you will have to deal with administrative complications that you really don't want to deal with when (and after) you have a baby.

In fact, around the sixth or seventh month is a good time to get the answers from your plan to a number of questions arising from delivery and beyond:

➤ How long is a hospitalization for a regular (vaginal) delivery? There is a law that allows at least 48 hours of hospitalization if you and your doctor agree, but you need to ask how it is calculated. If you are in labor for two hours, do you get to stay 46 more hours? The end of the next business day? If you're in labor 14 hours, do you get to stay another 34 hours?

➤ What are the health plan's guidelines for ordering a C-section? How long would you stay in the hospital after one?

➤ If you have to stay in the hospital and your baby doesn't, will the plan pay for the baby to stay? If not, what can the plan do to help your family through a difficult time?

169

➤ If the baby has to stay in the hospital and you don't, what should you expect? What are the arrangements for breastfeeding?

➤ Find out how, and how soon, you have to enroll the baby in the health plan as part of your family (see Chapter 7 for more on this). This is not automatic.

➤ Are home nursing visits part of the covered services? Can you opt for them? Can you get a deal on them? Home nursing visits can help you keep an eye on you and your newborn, and pick up any problems that may show up after you leave the hospital.

➤ What if you need special equipment at home? What is paid for and what is not?

➤ Some pediatric specialists have lactation consultants to assist with breastfeeding. These can include breast pump rentals. Ask the plan if they have lactation specialists as part of pediatric services.

➤ When must the baby be seen by the pediatrician after you go home? When must you be seen for a postpartum check-up?

What about a Cesarean, or C-section, delivery? A C-section is performed when the baby is taken from the mother's womb through an incision in the abdomen. Critics claim it is done much too often in this country and is needlessly risky to the mother with no benefit to the baby. But a C-section is necessary for either mother or child if a vaginal delivery is dangerous, the baby is in fetal stress, or a breech (feet-first) birth is impending. Find out what guidelines your plan uses, such as how often it is done, what indicates the need for a C-section, and when you have to make a decision on it. Talk to your obstetrician about your plan's approach for any added insight she has.

Be sure you pick a pediatrician ahead of time. Interview her as carefully as any other doctor (see Chapter 11). See if she can see the baby in the hospital. If there are problems, she will have some familiarity with her new little patient. Find out before you go to the hospital who to talk to if you have questions about the baby.

Your Personal Rx
Check with your plan about weight control programs after pregnancy, especially if you have a family history of diabetes. They are often offered by the plans and use nutritionists. With all the stresses on your body and your soul as a new mom, it's better to work on weight control with someone whose priority is health.

There are a few things you should do for yourself. If you plan to breastfeed, find out if your plan offers classes before your delivery and if they are given in the hospital. Make sure you schedule your postpartum physical. Make a list of questions you may have. It's also a good time to check out your plan's advice line, if you haven't done so already.

You can get bombarded by information in the hospital, with everything from poison center numbers to information about baby formula. Make sure you pick out checklists for baby care from your plan for emergency care and support lines and put those in a handy place at home.

And find a trusted mom. It always helps if you have someone nonjudgmental, with a sense of humor, whom you can ask what seem like very silly questions.

MC Moms: Managed Care Moms in Their Own Words

We talked to a lot of managed care moms (and that includes one of the authors) who shared their insights on what you should know.

One, a mother of three who had two miscarriages between her first two children, spoke eloquently of her hair-raising time in managed care. At the time, she belonged to a staff model HMO. The following suggestions for mothers-to-be spring from her own saga:

➤ Find out what is a pregnancy-related emergency to a managed care plan. When do you go to the emergency room, especially after office hours? Ask your obstetrician for guides on recognizing emergency situations. Ask your doctor who to call in certain situations. Is the advice line capable of handling maternity questions? How do you do this? Call with a couple trial questions.

➤ What do you do if you miscarry? Do you go to the ER? If you are bleeding, do you call an ambulance? "I may have handled my miscarriage differently if I had known what to expect, both of the plan and the ER," said our source.

➤ Make sure everyone involved—the mother, the ob-gyn, any attending doctors, and the plan—have their stories straight. Our source got conflicting information on what procedure she should have after the miscarriage.

Fast Action

The fourth pregnancy went fine, but the baby developed some skin abrasions that did not heal, and the plan would not refer the child to a specialist. Her approach now was the following:

➤ Ask what the plan considers an emergency. In this instance, the baby stopped eating at two weeks, cried continuously in pain, and began to lose weight.

➤ Get your advocates ready to act. She called a relative, who was an attorney, to write letters, overnight mailed to the health plan, including the head of pediatrics, demanding immediate referral out and threatening a lawsuit. The referral came.

At the university medical center, the doctors agreed with the health plan that the baby did not need a laser procedure. They did find that the baby had been misdiagnosed and mistreated in very basic medicine. The abrasion was finally treated as a burn, and, with attention to salve and wrappings, it healed. MC Mom and family incurred no costs.

The family switched medical plans (to a PPO) at the next open season. "My medical plan is worth more to me now than furniture for the house. That's where I'm going to invest," she said.

What MC Mom Wants and Gets

The new federal Newborns' and Mothers' Health Protection Act guarantees new moms the right to stay in the hospital for at least 48 hours if they and their doctor agree that it is useful. But little has been known about what managed care moms get, what they need, and how they feel about it. To remedy this lack, researchers surveyed over 5,000 female members of a large national managed care organization who had recently had a normal vaginal delivery. Some of their experiences and opinions might surprise you:

➤ The majority of moms in the northeast spent between one and two days in the hospital after delivery. The majority of moms in the rest of the country were out in a day or less.

➤ The majority of women who were in the hospital a day or less thought their stay was too short, while most of those who spent two days or more thought it was just about right. Overall, more than half of women thought their stay was too short.

➤ Spending less time in the hospital does not seem to be bad for the health of new moms and their babies. Women and their babies leaving the hospital in two days or less did not seem to be any more likely to be readmitted to the hospital than those staying longer. But some short-stay moms and their babies did have problems.

So what would make managed care moms happier?

➤ Regardless of how long they spent in the hospital, the majority of moms would have liked to get more information on caring for themselves and their babies after going home.

➤ Most women said they would be willing to go home within 24 hours after a future delivery, but many said they would want to do that only with additional services. Such services included access to a 24-hour hotline, a follow-up phone call by a health care professional, a home health visit, and housekeeping services.

If your plan has a policy of short maternity stays, find out what it is willing to offer in return. How about baby-care classes, especially for new parents? How about the 24-hour hotline? Some plans have them for all members. If yours doesn't, one for new moms (and dads!) would be appropriate. And if you're going to save the plan hundreds of dollars by giving up your room early, a home health visit isn't too much to ask for.

If you're planning to start a family, ask these questions when you are choosing a plan. The stork, we hear, doesn't always wait to visit until open season!

The Least You Need to Know

➤ Evaluate your plan and your obstetrician for the care you need. Know what your plan allows, how much it will cost, and if the obstetric care available is the care you want and need.

➤ Start prenatal visits as soon as you know you are pregnant. Make sure you ask about and understand any testing or procedure that may be done. Ask about the risks and the benefits.

➤ Be prepared to be an advocate for yourself and your baby. If yours is, or you believe it is, an at-risk pregnancy, make sure you understand the referral process. Line up your information and your allies.

➤ Know when you get to go home from the hospital, what happens if you or the baby needs to stay, and what help at home the plan might make available.

➤ Enjoy your baby. Eventually, they sleep through the night.

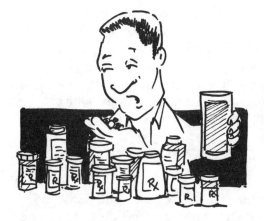

Living with It: Chronic Conditions

How healthy are you? Never better. Fit as a fiddle, except for a little arthritis in your shoulder after years of softball. Oh, and those migraines that hit once every couple months.

Surveys have found that about 9 in 10 people rate their health as "good" or better. Yet federal government data show that the average American has 1.7 *chronic conditions*. These conditions include things we rarely think about unless they get annoying, such as dry skin, hay fever, or the astigmatism that requires glasses. But they also include asthma, arthritis, diabetes, migraines, and heart problems, which can cause serious discomfort and even death unless they are treated on a continuing basis. And with recent advances in

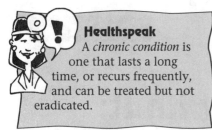

Healthspeak

A *chronic condition* is one that lasts a long time, or recurs frequently, and can be treated but not eradicated.

medical diagnosis and treatment, medical experts are even beginning to talk about conditions such as HIV/AIDS and cancer as "chronic."

Chronic disease is not for adults alone. About 20 million children have chronic diseases and disorders. These include asthma, juvenile diabetes, cerebral palsy, spina bifida, mental retardation, and cystic fibrosis, among others.

House Call

Seven diseases account for nearly half of the U.S. health bill: heart disease, cardiovascular disease, diabetes, cancer, arthritis, depression, and osteoporosis.

People with a chronic condition often don't "get better," despite medical treatment. Sometimes there are complicating factors, episodes of problems related to their disease. But with proper care and medical management, their lives can be pretty normal. This chapter tells you how to function as a chronic care patient in a managed care world.

Your Primary Care Doctor: First Among Equals

Don't expect to be cared for solely by a specialist. If you belong to a managed care plan, a good, competent primary care doctor is key to keeping you healthy.

Your primary care doctor is the coordinator of your care and often makes the principal decision to issue you a referral—your ticket—to specialist care (see Chapter 11 for more on this).

House Call

We use the term "primary care doctor" throughout the chapter. If you have a child with a chronic condition, just substitute "pediatrician." She's the primary care doctor for children.

The importance of picking a good primary care doctor was eloquently explained by Mike. Mike has belonged to HMOs for the past 13 years and has had colitis since he was 16. He belonged to a national HMO for eight years and a large, regional one for five. He is pleased with his care and gave us these bits of wisdom for choosing a primary care doctor:

"The most important thing to do is follow the rules. And pick a good gatekeeper, the primary care doctor. Gatekeepers are there for a reason; they are treating the whole person. Specialists respond to only one area. With a chronic disease like mine, communication is the key. Having a painful chronic condition is a very emotional experience. You have to listen hard, and they have to listen hard. Don't underestimate bedside manner. You have to feel free to talk. And if you are not happy with your specialist, tell your primary care doctor. Tell him you are unhappy, tell him why, and that you need to see someone else."

Many people with chronic illnesses told us to "go with your gut." Your number-one choice for primary care doctor must be someone you can talk to and someone you can trust. There will be a number of pushes and pulls on her from you, the managed care plan, her practice partners, and the hospital, if it becomes involved. You want someone who will be straight with you.

But it can be difficult to find a primary care doctor with knowledge of your condition. Your list of doctors in the directory most likely will not list the chronic illnesses with which their primary doctors have experience. Some doctors familiar with a disease or condition may have treated mostly males and few females, or vice versa. If you are part of an ethnic or racial group for whom some diseases are more likely to occur, finding the right primary care doctor can also be a problem.

Ask your current doctor or specialist if she is familiar with physicians on your new plan's list. Ask a local support group if they are familiar with any doctors on the list. And if you are joining an open network and you want to keep your current doctor, ask her if she would be able to join the plan. No harm in asking!

When you interview your new primary care doctor, ask how much experience she has with your condition. If you've had much experience with your own care, you'll get a sense of whether that doctor knows when to refer out. If you don't feel comfortable, find another candidate.

Whatever you do, don't postpone getting a primary care doctor when you join or change plans. Make it a number-one priority. If you don't, your ability to get good, continuous care could suffer.

Some Areas Are Best Left to Specialists

Whatever your plan, getting to a specialist has changed radically over the past ten years. You and your doctor are not the only ones involved, and it can get complicated, frustrating, and rule driven.

Here's a true story. A well-informed, savvy consumer had some scaly patches on her elbows that wouldn't go away. She, a non-physician, suspected psoriasis, a common skin condition. A member of a tightly managed HMO, she first saw her primary care doctor. The doctor agreed that it looked like psoriasis, but in her plan she had to see a dermatologist to have the diagnosis verified. Referral form in hand, she snagged the next available

177

appointment with the dermatologist—in three weeks. Two doctor visits and three weeks of ugly elbows later, the diagnosis was confirmed, and she got her prescription ointment. Twenty years ago, she would have gone to see one doctor—once—and the problem would already have been under control.

Some plans err on the side of generosity and others on the side of stinginess in administering specialist referrals. While stinginess is usually unpleasant, and can be downright damaging, generosity does not always serve the patient, either.

Your ability to consult the right specialist at the right time can mean the difference between life and death. People with chronic health conditions should be concerned about the same things as everyone else in choosing, using, and changing plans (see Chapters 1 through 7) but should consider the following additional questions as well.

Ask the Hard Questions

The checklist on the following page was created as a tool for those with HIV or AIDS choosing their health care plan. But it's also a great checklist to use whatever your chronic condition; just replace HIV/AIDS with the name of your condition.

Putting Their Tests to the Test

If your specialist suggests tests or procedures, especially if they are invasive, be aggressive. Sit down with him and ask questions that will unravel both the procedure and your plan's approach to your situation. Ask the following questions:

➤ What is he looking for in the tests (lab work or X rays or procedures)?

➤ How dangerous is it?

➤ Is it painful, and, if so, how is the pain managed? (This is particularly important if you are dealing with the after-care at home.)

➤ How long does it take, and how long does it take to recover?

➤ What are the potential risks for having it done, and what are the potential risks for not having it done?

If you are concerned about not having a particular test or procedure done, turn the questions listed above on their heads (that is, why not do test A, how can you find what you're looking for?). If you are really suspicious, ask if you would be treated differently if you had different insurance. They should be able to answer all these questions to your satisfaction.

If you are not satisfied, consider going outside the plan for a second opinion. You may be able to get the highest quality center for a diagnosis of your condition. You may want to get a second opinion from someone without a financial connection to your doctor or plan. As in other instances when you act on your own, be prepared to pay out-of-pocket, though your plan may pay.

Managed Care Checklist for People with HIV/AIDS (or Any Chronic Condition)

With earlier diagnosis and improvements in treatment, HIV/AIDS is becoming a long-term, chronic condition for many people. Here are some special managed care issues you should consider in choosing, using, and changing managed care plans. Most of these questions apply to both private plans and Medicaid managed care plans (see Chapter 10 for more on Medicaid):

❏ Does the plan contract with doctors, hospitals, and community-based health care providers with a track record of serving HIV/AIDS patients?

❏ Can I choose a physician with experience in HIV/AIDS as my primary care provider?

❏ Does the plan have a drug formulary (more on this later in this chapter)?

❏ If so, are off-label drugs (see Chapter 18) and new drugs for HIV/AIDS included in the formulary?

❏ How and how often is the formulary revised to include new and more effective drugs as they become available?

❏ How does the grievance/appeals process work (see Chapter 23)? How quickly are decisions made?

❏ What information does the plan have on the health outcomes of chronically ill people, including those with HIV/AIDS?

❏ What are the plan's policies on specialist referrals?

❏ What are the plan's policies on new HIV/AIDS drugs, new treatment protocols, and participation in clinical trials (see Chapter 18)?

❏ Many plans have consumer boards or advisory committees. If the plan has one, are people with HIV/AIDS and providers with HIV/AIDS expertise included?

Source: Adapted from AIDS Action Foundation, Medicaid Reform and Managed Care, undated.

Referrals

We interviewed lots of people for this book, and they told us that the most misunderstood rules, the source of the most contention, and the thing that gives the most hissy-fits to patients, lawyers, office staff, and doctors alike is referrals.

The whole referral process can be different from plan to plan. The ACHES Plan may allow six visits to a specialist before you need to return to your primary care doctor, while the PANES Plan may require a referral for each visit. There are few things as frustrating as relying on what you did in your last plan only to find out it gets you in trouble with your new one.

Make sure you understand what the referral means and how long you are able to use it. Is it one referral per specialist visit or is it for a series of visits? Find out how soon you have to use the referral once you have it and how often you can use it before you need another referral. Managed care plans often require that you go back to your primary care doctor when the referral needs to be renewed. This is part of their management technique, with the primary care doctor as the coordinator of your care.

When you look at that referral form, check the checks. Your doctor will have checked the boxes for when, how many visits, how long, and so on. If they are different from what you discussed in the office, march right back in and get the record straight.

Some managed care programs were reported to send children to adult specialists. In order to receive optimum care, children should go to pediatric specialists. Up to what age? It depends. One doctor told us of his patient, a 12-year-old boy recuperating from a compound fracture. He could have done fine with the orthopedists at the hospital where he initially went for treatment, but the doctor sent him to the local children's hospital because that hospital had specialists in administering anesthesia to children for the ensuing surgery.

Your Personal Rx

If you have children, find out if a managed care plan has pediatric specialists (and how many) before you join the plan. Even if your child doesn't need a specialist now, most likely he will need at least one referral before he is 18.

Referrals also cover tests. You need a referral (in some plans it's called a precertification) before any testing can be done. If your condition is not life threatening, any lab tests, X rays, or other tests may not be done immediately. Be sure you know if you are going to get that test right away or if the precertification or referral process is going to take a while. If it does, be prepared to follow up, and nudge it along if need be.

If your referrals have time limits or visit limits, make sure you get a new referral immediately after or just before the old one runs out. Don't wait until you have another episode requiring the specialist. One rheumatoid arthritis sufferer told us that he once had to have his lab tests postponed because he had waited too long to get the referral updated. Without the referral, the lab would not do the tests, even though he had been under treatment for more than a year.

Many managed care plans ration specialist referrals, but many of the large ones are coming to realize that getting the specialists involved sooner in the course of an illness saves money and improves patient outcomes.

If you want to see a specialist, or have been referred to one, see our checklists for obtaining and discussing specialty care in Chapter 17.

Prescription Drugs and Chronic Conditions

Twenty years ago, your ulcer may have been treated with surgery. Today, it may be treated with antibiotics. Advances in pharmaceuticals have changed the landscape of medical care. Treatment of chronic conditions often require long-term drug therapy, rather than invasive procedures requiring long hospital stays.

Some chronic conditions may not require any medication, may be treated satisfactorily with over-the-counter products, or may require a prescription drug only during an occasional flare-up, such as during allergy season. Other chronic conditions—diabetes, high blood pressure, or thyroid problems, for example—are managed, or treated, with prescription drugs on a long-term basis.

Big changes are afoot, and that means that you have to know something about how medications are handled in managed care plans.

So what's happened to your pharmacist? Even though the commercials prefer to high-light the friendly neighborhood pharmacist, eyeglasses off the bridge of his nose while he gently explains the prescription he has just filled, that role is ancient. Pharmacists are becoming administrators, whose role is to administer drug protocols and compliance programs. Technicians do the dispensing. Drug companies market their new products to managed care companies instead of physicians.

So before heading to the pharmacy, all health care consumers should be familiar with three terms:

➤ Formularies

➤ Generic substitution

➤ Therapeutic substitution

Many plans have adopted these techniques to reduce prescription drug costs. However, there are instances where improper savings on prescription drugs have led to preventable illnesses and even death. Here's what you need to know about the way managed care plans prescribe and pay for prescription drugs.

Formularies

Formularies—lists of prescription drugs a plan prefers for its enrollees—are typical among HMOs. While plans develop their formularies differently, the criteria for inclusion are typically safety, effectiveness, cost, and cost-effectiveness. Some plans also consider a drug's impact on a patient's quality of life (conve-nience and ability to carry on normal life activities) in their decisions. Plans may direct their formularies at doctors, pharmacists, plan members, or all three.

The impact of a formulary on the care *you* will receive will depend on both how restrictive the formulary is and how difficult it is to bypass. A formulary would generally not include all the drugs available and

Healthspeak

A *formulary* is a list of drugs or classes of drugs preferred by a health care plan for use by its enrollees. In an "open" formulary, the patient does not incur any financial penalties for using nonform-ulary drugs. In an "incentive-based" formulary, the patient pays a higher copayment for such drugs. In a "closed" formulary, nonformulary drugs are not covered at all.

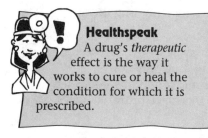

Healthspeak
A drug's *therapeutic* effect is the way it works to cure or heal the condition for which it is prescribed.

approved by the *Food and Drug Administration (FDA)* for a particular condition. Many prescription drugs are copies of each other; not all may need to be included. Many similar drugs, on the other hand, may have slightly different *therapeutic* (or curative) effects and side effects that can argue for the exclusion of some and the inclusion of others. However, patients, even with the same condition, are not all alike, and an extremely restrictive formulary could exclude products that would be the best choice for some patients.

If you have a chronic condition that is treated with one or more prescription drugs, let your new doctor know how you are doing on your current regimen as well as how you did on any drugs you may have tried previously for the same condition. If your doctor wants you to try something different from what you are taking, ask why. Even if your previous treatment has been successful, your new doctor may know about ways to treat you with a lower dosage or fewer side effects, or at a lower cost.

Many doctors participate in dozens of managed care plans. Most won't remember what each plan's formulary includes. To save time, many may use the most restrictive formulary of the plans they belong to in writing prescriptions. Always ask if a particular drug your doctor is prescribing is the best and most modern drug for your condition, especially if you have had good experience with another product.

Healthspeak
The *Food and Drug Administration (FDA)* is a federal agency that evaluates and approves prescription drugs. Drugs are usually approved for treating a particular illness or injury but may later be found useful in treating additional conditions. Whether or not they have a formulary, plans typically exclude coverage for such "off-label" uses unless the drug's effectiveness in such uses has been documented in published research.

If you are in a plan with a formulary, the doctor might not prescribe the drug you would like, or are used to, unless you ask. If the formulary is open or incentive-based, you should be able to get the drug you want as long as your doctor approves and you are willing to pay any additional copayment that may apply. In a plan with a closed formulary, the doctor may need to obtain prior authorization to have a nonformulary drug covered.

If you are in a plan that uses a formulary, you may not have prompt access to all new drugs. In one study of managed care plans, more than half of the plans studied assessed at least half of all new drugs for inclusion in their formularies, but that still leaves a lot of drugs out of a lot of plans. Not having access to all new drugs may not hurt your health, because some new drugs are simply copies of drugs already on the market. But if you have a condition with few effective standard treatments, you should make sure you are aware of any drugs that represent true advances, because your plan may not inform you.

If authorization for a nonformulary drug is not granted, you may need to file an appeal, enter into arbitration, or even go to court to obtain coverage (more on this in Chapters 23 and 24). This course of action may make sense if the drug you need is too expensive to afford on your own.

Because appeals, arbitration, and litigation can take a long time, however, you should try to see if you can obtain a supply of the drug while your case is pending. Otherwise, your health could deteriorate during the time it takes to get your plan's approval. First, see if the drug's manufacturer will provide you with a supply. Many have hardship programs that could apply in your case. Second, see if there are any clinical trials using the drug that you might be qualified to enter (more on advanced treatments in Chapter 18). Finally, find out if you might qualify for coverage through a state prescription drug program. Your state's insurance commissioner, department of public health, or department of social services should be able to help.

What's in a Name: Generic Substitution

When a company first invents a new prescription drug, it has a period of time under which the drug's formula is protected by patent. Once the patent expires, other companies can make the same drug, using the same formula; they just can't call it the same thing. The copy is called the "generic." It usually sells for much less than the original "branded" drug, though some managed care plans that buy very large quantities may be able to get better prices on the branded drug than on the generic. Many of the "house brands" of food or toiletries you may buy in your supermarket are applications of the same "copycat" concept.

Healthspeak
Generic substitution is the replacement of a prescription drug with another product containing the same active ingredient in the same amount and dosage form, but sold by a different company. All states have laws permitting generic substitution.

Your doctor will usually note on your prescription whether the pharmacist is authorized to substitute a generic form of the drug if one is available. If you have been taking a brand name and the generic is authorized (or the other way around), ask why. Sometimes even two drugs that are chemically identical may be used differently by the body. If you are changing between the brand and generic versions of a prescription drug, ask what side effects you may expect to encounter.

Therapeutic Substitution: Even Your Doctor May Not Know for Sure

Many large hospitals and HMOs allow their pharmacists to substitute entirely different drugs for drugs prescribed by doctors, so long as the substituted drug is of the same pharmacological or therapeutic class. This practice is called *therapeutic substitution*. The substitution is usually made from the hospital or HMO's formulary, which, in turn, has been evaluated on behalf of the hospital or plan.

Healthspeak
Therapeutic substitution is the replacement of a prescribed drug with an entirely different drug of the same pharmacological or therapeutic class. Most state laws are silent on therapeutic substitution.

Your Personal Rx
If your doctor has bad handwriting, ask him or her to spell clearly for you the name of any drug you are being told to take.

Your Personal Rx
If you have a chronic condition that may render you unconscious or unable to respond, wear a Medic Alert bracelet. You can get one at your local pharmacy.

Therapeutic substitution poses significantly more danger than generic substitution. Various drugs, even those in a single class, may have different biological effects, side effects, and interactions. For example, while both aspirin and ibuprofen are both nonsteroidal anti-inflammatory drugs, aspirin reduces the blood's ability to clot, while ibuprofen does not.

While pharmacists should inform doctors of therapeutic substitutions, they do not always do so. When you receive a new prescription, make sure you understand what it is, as well as any discrepancies between what was prescribed and what you actually get.

Emergencies

One of the problems common to chronic conditions is knowing when an episode is acute or mild, and what to do about these different types of episodes. That's why communication with both your specialist and your primary care doctor is so important, especially if acute episodes can land you in the ER.

If you or a family member have a chronic health condition, make sure you have a checklist handy of the types of episode that will require emergency care and the types that won't. Your doctor should be able to provide you with one. Talk it over with both your primary care doctor and your specialist. Make sure someone else who is often with you knows where the list is, or even has a copy. Sometimes they are the ones who have to make the decision.

If you call the urgent care line, tell them immediately that you have a specific condition, you are under treatment, and list the medications you are taking. (See Chapter 14 for more details on what to do in emergency situations.)

Disease Management Programs

If you have a chronic condition such as asthma, diabetes, or arthritis, you should ask your plan's advice line or member services department whether you are eligible to participate in a *disease management* program. Don't be surprised, actually, if in many large plans the disease management program finds you!

How does disease management differ from the way patients have been treated in the past? Instead of focusing on the individual components of the disease, it focuses on the whole patient.

What is included in a disease management program can differ widely among plans, as can the way the program is structured. Some programs are largely long-term monitored drug treatment, without other components such as patient education or behavior modification. Some plans assign patients who have particular conditions such as asthma or diabetes to a case manager, who may have the authority to go beyond plan provisions to combine health care resources to fit the patient's needs. Disease management programs may also add patient education, an important component in the management of conditions in which patient compliance with treatment regimens and other health habits has an important impact on outcomes. (See Chapter 12 for more on preventive care.)

The major conditions for which disease management programs have been developed include:

➤ Arthritis

➤ Asthma

➤ Cancer

➤ Congestive heart failure

➤ Depression

➤ Diabetes

➤ High blood pressure

➤ High cholesterol

➤ HIV/AIDS

➤ Osteoporosis

People with chronic health conditions should be aware that separate, specialized providers of disease management programs are being hired by managed care plans. Managed care networks have long contracted with specialized providers of mental health and substance abuse treatment (more on this in Chapter 19). Similar specialized providers are emerging for such conditions as cancer and diabetes. If you and your doctors decide that such a specialized program is for you, make sure your primary care doctor remains informed about your progress and needs. Extra attention to one aspect of your health should not cause other aspects to fall through the cracks.

Healthspeak

A *case management program* provides comprehensive health care services tailored to the patient's needs. *Case managers* are usually allowed to provide services not usually covered under the plan, or in settings that may not usually be covered, such as the patient's home, if deviating from the plan's rules meets the patient's needs better.

The Best Advocate You Can Be

You may never need to be an advocate. Your specialist and primary care physician may be in the same building, understand each other's instructions completely, and your plan may never question any decision you or your doctors make. Your doctors may stay with the plan for the rest of your life. You may never, ever forget, misread, or lose your referral form. But if this scenario is not true, be prepared to be your own best advocate.

Start preparing even before you join a plan. When choosing an HMO, check your access to specialists, the board certifications of participating doctors, the location of its clinics, the ease of getting appointments, and if it has a 24-hour advice line. If you check this out before joining and your expectations are not met, seriously consider changing plans when you have a chance.

You also need to know your disease or condition. Join the national organization (almost all diseases have one) for reliable information about your disease and the latest treatments. Go to local support group meetings and lectures for good updates and coping strategies. Trading experiences, including experiences with specific managed care plans, can be extremely valuable.

Especially be prepared if you are an "outlier," that is, your condition takes a different course from that of most people with the disease. It could be more or less severe than that of the typical patient, or could proceed more quickly or more slowly. This is where you really have to know how to manage the managers.

Your Personal Rx
We asked our friend with Crohn's disease what people should keep in mind as they work on a treatment plan outside the norm. He said, "Remember that the specialists and primary care doctors are the experts on how to get through the bureaucracy. Use them whenever you can." That's good advice for anyone with a chronic condition.

Be prepared to do your own research. One patient with Crohn's disease told us that he found his HMO is good at keeping current, but they don't like extreme treatment. If you want treatment other than what they do for the majority of patients who have your particular disease, figure out what outcome you want and how you are going to get there.

Be prepared to negotiate. Find out the best possible and worst possible outcomes and the normal outcome for each level of decision you and your treatment team need to make. Because the patient with Crohn's disease wanted to avoid surgery until he had a bad test, his doctors had to justify that course of treatment. His way could raise the costs for the HMO. His latest HMO had him work out what he would do when he had to make a decision about surgery.

The Least You Need to Know

➤ If your doctor asks you to change from a drug that you have used successfully for your condition, ask why and what side effects you can expect from the change. If you don't understand or don't agree with the answers to these questions, ask to stay on your old prescription.

➤ Finding a good, knowledgeable primary care doctor or pediatrician is especially important for those with chronic conditions. If you join or change managed care plans, make picking a new primary care physician a number-one priority.

➤ Know your disease. Learn what to expect, when an episode is mild or acute, and what its course is likely to be.

➤ Know how your plan's referrals work. This is one of the most frustrating parts of managed care, and one that can impact your health severely.

➤ Be prepared to be an advocate for yourself. Sometimes that means challenging the system. Sometimes it means negotiating to get the treatment you want.

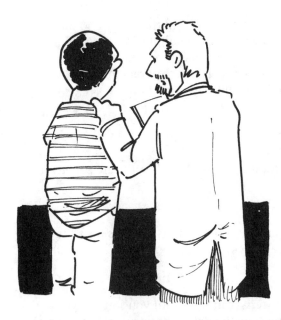

Chapter 17

When the Unexpected Happens: Injuries and Illness

In This Chapter
➤ Getting second (and third) opinions
➤ Deciding if a specialty center is right for you
➤ Discussing specialty treatment with your doctors
➤ Making your case when you disagree

If you're old enough, you probably remember exactly where you were and what you were doing when you heard about the assassination of President John F. Kennedy or the explosion of the Challenger space shuttle. Many people who have ever had a serious illness have the same vivid memory of the day the doctor told them something was wrong. Your whole view of the world can change; the earth seems to wobble on its axis.

A major illness or injury can require specialty care. Unfortunately, many people need to think about specialty care at some point in their lives. Some may even want to explore treatments medical science is only beginning to learn about (read about those in Chapter 18).

This chapter and the one following are intended to take some of the worry and uncertainty out of serious illnesses or injuries and may even save your life. We can't bring you chicken soup and fluff your pillows, but we will help you make the health care system work for you when it really matters. You are facing paperwork requirements you may have never seen before, and we will walk you through them. (And you can get good chicken soup in a can!)

Get That Second Opinion!

You've just had bad news. Not the time you want to think about health care paperwork, right?

Wrong!

This is *exactly* the time when health care paperwork really matters. (Unless it's a life-threatening emergency; in that case, read Chapter 14, on emergency care, and let the paperwork wait.)

Before you do anything else, get a second, and even a third, opinion. And we mean *anything* else. Most conditions—even most cancers—can wait until you sort out your options. (If your doctor says you can't wait, he could be right, but you should ask why.)

Many people facing a serious health problem are afraid to get a second opinion for fear of insulting their doctor. Don't be! Doctors we interviewed for this book *want* you to get another opinion. Doing so can help you and your doctor understand your problem better, open up new treatment options, and even help your recovery. Even if you remember nothing else from reading this book, remember to get a second opinion any time you are confronted with bad health news.

House Call

People who are actively engaged in their treatment recover better from a serious illness—and live longer—than those who are not. Accept all the help you can get. If you have a choice, delegate away tasks at home or work rather than interactions with your plan and doctors. Someone who is unfamiliar with your plan can miss things that you would catch.

What Went Wrong

There are two points at which you should get a second opinion: the diagnosis (what's wrong) and the treatment (what to do about it). Many people skip the first step. Bad news is so upsetting, most people just want to be cured as soon as possible. But you should get a second opinion on the diagnosis, especially if your condition is potentially life-threatening or calls for invasive procedures such as surgery.

The first and second opinions often disagree, even on the diagnosis. For example, even experienced specialists may confuse some types of cancer with precancerous abnormalities. In that case, get a third opinion, ask the first two practitioners to resolve their differences, or see if you can refer the first two opinions to a specialist at a university, who may deal extensively with confusing or unusual cases.

Managed care plans differ in their second opinion requirements:

➤ Some plans require a second opinion before authorizing surgery. Use this safety net thoughtfully to get the best advice you can; don't just look at it as another hurdle to clear before signing into the hospital.

➤ Some plans cover the cost of a second opinion only if it is rendered by another physician in the network. That's better than nothing, but may not give you access to the expert advice you want.

➤ Some plans won't cover the cost of a second opinion at all. You should pay for it yourself if you have to; after all, you have set up your rainy day fund, or your flexible spending account if you are eligible, haven't you? See Chapter 5 for more on flexible spending accounts and setting up a rainy day fund.

Choose an expert for the second opinion. One patient first diagnosed with early-stage breast cancer took her slides to a well-known cancer research center for a second opinion. The slides were read by a medical resident—a student, not an experienced specialist—who thought the slides showed widespread cancer. That would have suggested a mastectomy, or removal of the breast. Several weeks of unnecessary stress later, the conflict in diagnoses was resolved, and the patient had a lumpectomy—breast-sparing surgery—instead.

> **Your Personal Rx**
> If your plan doesn't cover the cost of a second opinion and you are worried about it, *ask the doctor giving the second opinion.* The second opinion should usually cost no more than the average doctor's appointment in your area.

What to Do About It

If your diagnosis is confirmed, get a second opinion on the treatment. Medicine is still an art as much as a science. First and second opinions, therefore, differ a surprising amount of the time.

Despite managed care's emphasis on avoiding unnecessary surgery, many doctors still think of surgery first. Even if both opinions agree, you may want to look at a

> **Caution**
> If your first opinion suggests surgery but the second does not, your plan may require you to get a third opinion before authorizing surgery.

surgery recommendation very carefully. After all, once something is taken out, they can't put it back in! Ask about alternatives to surgery:

➤ One patient with fibroid tumors (nonmalignant tumors of the uterus) talked her doctors out of a hysterectomy *twice*, opting for less-radical fibroid removal each time. The key in her case was a referral to another doctor in the same plan.

➤ One patient with painful arthritis of the neck was offered surgery but was pain free after six weeks of chiropractic therapy combined with easy at-home stretching exercises.

➤ You may want to leave town, at least for a consultation, if you don't want the surgery being offered to you. Researchers have found huge variations among regions of the country, from city to city, and even in adjacent small towns in the rates at which certain surgical procedures are performed. These variations are so large they can't be explained by geographic differences in health. They suggest that medical practice styles vary widely, and you may be able to get the treatment you want by shopping around.

House Call

Regional variations in medical practices can vary dramatically. One study found that 44 percent of women diagnosed with early-stage breast cancer in a recent year underwent mastectomies (removal of the breast). But this percentage varied from a low of 29 percent in Connecticut to a high of 58 percent in New Mexico. Similarly, many older men develop a benign form of prostate disease. The chances that a man will undergo prostate surgery by age 85 range from 15 percent in some communities to over 50 percent in others. Yet early surgery appears to lead to a slight *decrease* in life expectancy because this form of prostate disease does not become life-threatening for most men.

Referrals, Again

"Referral" can mean one or both of two things in managed care. The first meaning is the same as in any other type of plan: Your doctor makes a recommendation for further care. Most competent doctors know when they are out of their league, and if you followed our guidelines in Chapter 11, you selected a competent doctor. So start by asking your doctor if you should see a specialist, and if so, who.

The second meaning is unique to managed care plans: It's an authorization by the plan to see someone other than your primary care doctor. Both the doctor and the plan may have to sign off on a referral. Depending on how your doctor is paid by your plan, excessive referrals may be charged against her income for the year. But if she is reluctant to refer you to a specialist, it could be because she feels she can treat your condition equally well. Go through our checklist below for discussing specialty care with her and see how you feel about the answers you get.

Some plans contract with one or a few specialty providers for certain types of care. For example, if you need radiation treatment for cancer, your plan may contract with only one hospital. Your choice of specialist may then be limited to those who practice at that hospital. HMOs are especially likely to work this way. It's still important for you to be comfortable with the doctor treating you, so ask to change doctors, even within that group, if you feel you need to.

Some plans require that all decisions made by the specialist be cleared with the primary care doctor, or even a nurse employed by the plan. Decisions subject to such clearances could include adding extra radiation sessions or follow-up treatment for a cancer patient. Such clearances can ensure continuity, coordination, and communication with respect to your care. But such requirements may also mean that the primary care physician is being asked to sign off on treatments he does not understand.

Your Personal Rx
One specialist suggested the following specialist-selection technique. If you have, for example, a heart problem, call the cardiac ward of the nearest hospital and ask a nurse for his or her recommendations. Nurses *know*.

Caution
Schedule your specialist appointments carefully. In many managed care plans, referrals are good for only a short period of time, and you must have your referral in hand for the plan to cover the appointment.

Onerous clearance and approval requirements can affect your health, some specialists told us. A patient in a plan with such requirements may not get referred for specialized or advanced treatments as easily (more on advanced treatments in Chapter 18). If your plan has such requirements, you can stack the odds in your favor by taking the initiative to keep your primary care doctor in the loop. Ask your specialist such questions as:

➤ What happens next?

➤ Do you need to call someone?

➤ Should I make the call/pick up or send the records/draft the letter?

House Call

Even in an urban area, your plan's specialty doctor or hospital may be a long commute away. If the treatment is daily or long term—for example, physical therapy or radiation treatment—your plan may approve treatment by a provider closer to you. But be careful; the contract provider may be better. Ask your doctor to advise you and intervene with the plan if necessary.

When Is a Specialty Center Right for You?

It's only natural to look for the best care and best facilities when faced with a medical problem. When should you consider specialty centers for your care?

Kids Are Not Small Adults

Children have different medical needs than adults. All the doctors we interviewed agreed that children with major illnesses or injuries should be treated by pediatric specialists in the treatment of that illness or injury.

If there is a children's hospital in your area, most of the pediatric specialists in your area probably have privileges (are allowed to admit patients) there. But not all do. If you are interested in a specialist who does not have children's hospital privileges, balance the pros and cons carefully, with your doctor's help.

How Special?

If you have a rare, unusual condition, you might be well advised to consult a specialist or a specialty institution, wherever that may take you. Your doctor(s), the faculty of the nearest medical school, or Internet sites dealing with your condition can help you find a referral.

But, depending on your condition, there may be different levels of specialization and proficiency even in your own community. Your doctor(s) should know which local hospitals do most of the procedures you may need and which specialists do best with your condition. You may also be able to find Internet information comparing your plan's hospital(s) with others in your area (more on this in Chapter 6).

Sometimes your best option may be a hospital affiliated with a medical school or research center with specialists in your condition. But remember, be an informed consumer, not a starry-eyed consumer. Some academic and research hospitals do path-breaking work in their fields, but that may not be what you need.

And academic hospitals can carry certain drawbacks from the ordinary patient's standpoint. You may be treated by medical students or by fellows (newly minted docs) much of the time. Most doctors who are practicing medicine will admit they know more—even after only a few years of practice—than they did as students or fellows. And even the specialists who treat you may not be like the doctors you are used to seeing. People choose a career in medical research because research—not treating patients—is what they want to do. Would you feel better with a doctor who sees patients 12 months a year (okay, 11—take a vacation, doc), or one who sees them two months a year? If your condition and the available treatment indicates an academic hospital, go for it—but with your eyes wide open.

Remember, too, that there are ways to get the best of both worlds. You might want to go to an academic medical specialist for a second opinion, a consultation, or a treatment plan, but remain under the long-term care of your own doctor. Ask questions and find the mix that works best for you.

Sometimes Bigger Is Just...Bigger

Practice makes perfect. That's true whether you are trying to do the perfect dive or the perfect heart surgery. That's why we consult specialists and specialty institutions.

But for any specialty or procedure, bigger is not always better. Hospitals that do more of a particular surgery often have higher death rates. Hospitals that specialize in a particular condition or procedure will attract the most difficult-to-treat patients, who may have the lowest chance of survival in the first place. These patients will make the hospital's death rate higher than it would be if it treated only the healthier prospects. Statisticians attempt to adjust death rates to account for how sick the patients were when they came in the door, but these methods may not be fully accurate.

One specialist suggested to us, however, that after a certain point, a hospital's size may work against the patient. In a very large hospital, patients may be treated by physician assistants or medical students, or simply "fall through the cracks." So if you and your doctor(s) agree that a specialty institution is best for you, a mid-sized center may give you the mix of experience and personal attention that will speed your recovery.

How to Talk About It

You've just had a scary diagnosis. You're sitting in an office papered floor to ceiling with diplomas. Can't you relax and let the doctor tell you what to do?

Not yet.

Ask your doctor a few questions. The answers may make you feel better about your prospects—or send you in search of another doctor.

Your Specialty Treatment Checklist

❏ Do you and the doctor "click?" Do you feel comfortable asking questions? Does the doctor ask *you* questions, or is he proceeding on the basis of assumptions about you that may not be valid?

❏ *Don't panic* just because someone in a white coat suggests surgery. Even in a managed care plan, doctors may be too quick to recommend certain types of surgeries. In particular, ask a lot of questions if your doctor recommends a hysterectomy, prostatectomy, back surgery, or gall bladder removal, surgeries that are commonly overused.

❏ If either your doctor or your own research suggests that you have more than one option (surgery or none; major surgery or less major), ask your doctor to compare the costs, both to you and to the plan. Your doctor may be under pressure from your plan to recommend the option that costs the plan the least, even if the higher-cost option is better for you. In other cases, the doctor's fee for a simpler and a more complex surgery may be equal. The plan's fee structure could bias your doctor's recommendation to you.

❏ Find out how much experience your doctor has had in treating your condition. People with lots of successful experience *love* to talk about it! Remember that even surgeons, who are specialists themselves, may specialize in different parts of the body. For a simple or common surgery, a general surgeon may be as good a choice as a specialist. For a more difficult case, however—such as a rare or large tumor—you may want to insist on a specialist.

❏ Ask if the recommended treatment (drugs, surgery, physical therapy, or rehabilitation) will solve your problem or just alleviate the symptoms. If it's only the latter, think about the most conservative treatment options—diet modification, physical therapy, or chiropractic treatments, to name a few—first.

❏ If the treatment will involve surgery or a hospital stay, where does the doctor have privileges? Do you want to go to that hospital? Is the hospital one of your contract hospitals? If not, is the doctor willing to help you convince your plan to approve treatment there? If you want an exception to a plan rule, the plan is more likely to listen to your doctor than to you. If your doctor has had bad experiences in trying to convince your plan to approve exceptions, or shows a disinclination to do so for other reasons, find a doctor with privileges at a participating hospital. You don't need the stress!

❏ What can you expect during treatment or after surgery? Can you expect to feel pain, tired, depressed, more hungry, or less hungry than usual?

When the Care You Get Is Not the Care You Want

After you go through all these steps, you might still have doubts about the diagnosis, the proper treatment, who should deliver it, or who should pay for it. You're still in charge.

As we've been telling you throughout this book, plans have formal procedures for appealing treatment or reimbursement decisions (covered in Chapter 23). Or you may need to go to court (covered in Chapter 24). But these procedures are cumbersome, may not always get you the result you want, and may not even be necessary.

Before bringing out the heavy artillery, make sure you are not missing any obvious problems that are easy to solve. Run through the following checklists.

Checklist for Getting a Specialist Referral

❏ If you are having trouble getting your primary care doctor or plan to authorize a referral to a specialist, try to provide additional evidence. Have you explained everything, such as what, when, and where the problem is? Chart your symptoms to see if there are patterns: Do you get better after you eat or worse at night? Here's where your Internet access fee may pay for itself: You may be able to use your computer to seek out research evidence to make your case or help your doctor do so.

❏ Ask to see your medical records. They could be incomplete or contain errors that affect decisions about your treatment. This is especially likely if you have changed plans or your doctor left your plan and all your records did not make the trip with you.

❏ Ask to see another doctor in your plan. Even partners in the same group practice may have different experience, perspectives, and practice patterns.

❏ There is nothing new under the sun. There could be discussion or support groups dealing with your medical condition in your community. People there may have faced the same problem you have and coped with it successfully.

❏ If you feel the problem is too urgent to wait for a response to a letter or phone call, write anyway and consult a specialist at your own expense. If the specialist finds a problem that is covered under your plan, the plan is probably obligated to treat you for it or pay for the treatment you have obtained on your own, and you have left a paper trail that shows you wanted to do the right thing.

Checklist for Talking to Your Plan About Anything

❏ Call or write the insurance company's or managed-care plan's medical director or member services department. Explain your problem logically and briefly. Explain what you want and whom you've already asked for it. Get the name of the person on the other end of the line. Make notes on the points you want to make before you call and work from this "script." It may feel awkward at first, but a script helps keep you calm and focused on the facts in a difficult situation and can prevent the need for follow-up calls.

❏ If you write, make sure the letter is coherent and understandable to someone who does not know the problem from scratch. If the issue is complex and emotionally charged, ask someone whose judgment you trust to see if the letter gives enough information on its own for the plan's utilization reviewers to make a decision. But if you are filing a formal appeal, your letter should probably be written by an attorney (see Chapter 23).

❏ In some cases, including a chronology (what happened first, what happened next, who said what when it happened) in your explanation is important, but don't make it of the "he said, she said" variety. Capture the main events. After all, you're keeping a health diary anyway (either on tape or in writing), aren't you?

❏ If you write to your plan or insurance company, send a copy of the letter to the plan's state regulators (see Chapter 25) and note on the letter that you are doing this.

❏ If you call, you may not need to write. But if you write, call, too. The reason is that nobody *has* to respond to a letter; it can get shuffled from inbox to inbox. If you call, on the other hand, someone has to take the time to talk to you.

❏ Try not to call when you are frightened, confused, or fuming over the incompetence of the doctor, hospital, or pharmacy. Cool down first.

❏ Don't just demand or complain, and *never* threaten. Do you like to deal with people like that? Or do you prefer to deal with people who treat you with courtesy and respect? People who are perceived as cranks don't get a fair hearing but can get a psychiatric referral (this really happens!). More importantly, you're probably not threatening the person(s) with the power to help you.

❏ Speaking of help, take advantage of what may be available. Your doctor's office may not be a participating provider in your plan but may be willing to file your claim or investigate your benefits anyway. The office staff may know how to ask better questions than you do.

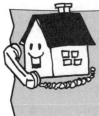

House Call

In some states, your doctor can pass on to your next doctor or plan only those records that were generated in your first doctor's office. If you have had a long and exciting medical history, keep track of all the installments yourself, or they could be lost to history.

Time Is Money

It can also mean your health. Many plans take their time in responding to your queries about reimbursement denials. Run out the clock, and your rights are gone.

When you are mailing a claim or questioning the plan's decision about treatment or payment, make a note on your calendar ("Sent in claim on Junior's knee injury" is enough.) Follow up if you have not heard in a reasonable period of time, usually two to three weeks at most. And when you talk to a representative of the plan or insurance company, ask, "When can I call you for the check/referral/decision?" Then put it on your calendar and do it.

Your Personal Rx

If all else fails, pay for your treatment yourself if you can, or try to talk the doctor or hospital into treating you on credit. In addition to protecting your health, you may be protecting important legal rights to reimbursement from your plan (see Chapter 23).

If you have applied our checklist and still aren't happy, you may need to file a formal appeal with your plan. Skip ahead to Chapters 23 and 24.

The Least You Need to Know

➤ If you're confronted with bad health news, get a second opinion on both the diagnosis and the treatment.

➤ If your doctor suggests surgery, ask about and read up on alternatives. There could be many.

➤ The best specialty treatment for you could be across town—or across the country. Make your decision based on the evidence and the advice of people and sources you trust.

➤ If you have trouble getting a referral you think you need or a reimbursement you think you are entitled to, see if the problem can be resolved by presenting more evidence, either to your doctor or to the plan.

➤ If the problem can't wait, pay for the test or treatment yourself or try to get it on credit. You could be protecting not only your health but also important legal rights.

➤ If nothing in this chapter works and you still think you're right, you may need to file a formal appeal or even go to court.

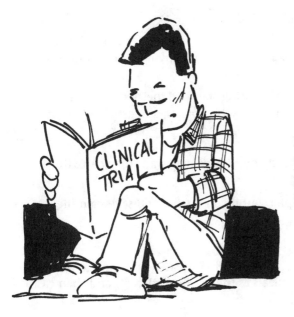

Chapter 18

More Than Standard Treatment

In This Chapter

➤ Deciding what's "experimental"

➤ Figuring if a clinical trial is right for you

➤ Talking to people who know

➤ Making sure someone else pays

This chapter is about the frontiers of medicine. These frontiers can be just as wild and woolly as the American West of yore. You can find

➤ Outlaws (purveyors of useless treatments) lurking in the shadows

➤ Lots of fighting (medicines and treatments against disease; maybe you and your doctor against your health care plan)

➤ Lawmen (maybe regulators, maybe your doctor or other trusted source of information, maybe your lawyer) dedicated to keeping order

We wrote this chapter for two groups of people:

➤ People for whom conventional treatments have not worked. For example, sometimes cancer doesn't respond to the surgery-chemotherapy-radiation routine—or seems to and then comes back.

➤ People whose conditions are not treatable using standard methods, or conditions that standard medicine can treat—diabetes, cystic fibrosis, and arthritis, to name a few—but not cure.

If you fit into either of these groups, you and your doctor may want to explore the frontiers of medicine.

We hope you never have to read this chapter. But if you do, it could save your life.

Is It Experimental?

We don't know about you, but our idea of "experiments" is based on long-ago high-school science courses. We combined chemicals as the teacher ordered...and then cleaned up the resulting mess.

Are you afraid of becoming a guinea pig (a perfectly nice little animal) and being subjected to the mercies of frowning people in white lab coats? Relax. The part about the lab coats is true, but that's only so you'll be able to tell the medical staff from the pizza delivery man. The rest isn't.

Experimental or investigational treatments have typically been tested extensively before being offered to patients. Indeed, many treatments and procedures are continuously evolving. For example, cancer treatment professionals are constantly evaluating how much—or how little—of a drug patients need to show improvement. Likewise, in the years that oral contraceptives have been available, research has dramatically decreased their hormonal content. In both cases, reducing the amount of drugs administered—while maintaining their clinical effectiveness—has reduced unwanted, and sometimes serious, side effects. So, really, all medicine, to some extent, is experimental.

But to keep its costs down—and to protect your health—your health care plan will want to draw the line somewhere. Here are several red flags managed care plans and others use to identify experimental or investigational treatments they won't pay for:

➤ There is inadequate published, scientific evidence to substantiate the treatment's safety or effectiveness in treating the illness or injury involved.

➤ If the treatment is effective, it is not at least as effective as any standard or established treatment.

➤ Benefits achieved in the trial can't be duplicated in an ordinary doctor-patient setting.

➤ In the case of a prescription drug or medical device, the U.S. Food and Drug Administration has not approved the product for marketing.

➤ Anybody with the authority to say so (generally a professional society or research facility) has determined that the treatment is experimental or investigational.

Your Personal Rx

If a medical practitioner offers you a drug or treatment that has *never* been tried before, run in the opposite direction, especially if he or she can't or won't answer the questions posed in this chapter.

Clinical Trials

In thinking about various experimental, investigational, or advanced treatment options, you may find it useful to distinguish among controlled experiments, or what researchers call "two-armed" studies, and treatments that have already been established to work in selected patients. In a two-armed study, one "arm" or group of patients receives the experimental treatment, while the other receives either standard treatment or no treatment. The progress of the two groups is then monitored to determine which alternative is best. In such a study, you run the risk of being put into the group receiving standard treatment, but you should never be put into a group getting *no* treatment if an established treatment for your condition exists.

Clinical trials are two-armed studies that explore new methods or materials, such as prescription drugs, new procedures, or new ways of using known materials, in the treatment of a disease or condition. Clinical trials are carefully controlled and managed to both help participants and expand medical knowledge, while keeping risks to patients as low as possible. Usually people will want to participate in a trial if it deals with a condition they have or, sometimes, fear they might develop.

Some perfectly healthy people may be interested in participating as well. If you are one of these people, you usually get a modest stipend or some other incentive such as a free medical check-up. The incentive for healthy people to participate (in addition to the money or other goodies) is generally the chance to see medical research from the inside and perhaps contribute to the resolution of a medical problem. Patients are seen regularly to determine the effect of the treatment, and treatment is always stopped if the side effects are too severe.

Healthspeak

A *clinical trial* is an investigation of new methods, materials, or procedures in the treatment of a particular disease or condition. Clinical trials may study ways to prevent, detect, diagnose, control, and treat various diseases, as well as the psychological impact of the diseases and ways to improve the patient's comfort and quality of life.

Clinical trials of new prescription drugs typically proceed in three phases:

➤ In Phase I, researchers test the safety of the drug in people. Patients are not accepted into Phase I trials if there are any proven or standard treatments for their condition, because the efficacy of Phase I drugs in human beings has not yet been established. Patients are carefully monitored for adverse effects. The advantage to the patient of participating in a Phase I trial is that if the drug turns out to be effective, the patient may have had access to it years before it becomes widely available. The disadvantage, of course, is that the drug may turn out to be useless. About 70 percent of experimental drugs pass this phase.

➤ If Phase I trials establish a drug's safety, researchers may proceed to Phase II, in which the drug's effectiveness is tested. If you have cancer that no longer responds to standard therapy, you may be a good candidate for a Phase II trial. The impact of the drug is compared with standard treatments, if available, or with a placebo (sugar pill) treatment if no standard treatment is available. About one-third of experimental drugs pass both Phase I and Phase II.

➤ In Phase III, researchers obtain a more thorough understanding of the drug's effectiveness, benefits, and range of possible adverse reactions. You can expect to be one of tens, hundreds, or thousands of participants. If the drug passes this test, as a rule, it becomes standard treatment.

House Call

Participants in clinical trials are *never* given a placebo or no treatment if there is an effective standard treatment available for their condition. The idea is that participating in a clinical trial should never make you worse off than if you had continued standard treatment.

Phase III trials are usually double-blind; this means neither the investigator nor the patient knows who gets the experimental treatment. This information is kept by an outside research group that acts as a storehouse for information on the study.

Checklist for Evaluating a Clinical Trial

The National Cancer Institute suggests that you ask the questions listed in the following table if you are considering taking part in a clinical trial. While the questions are designed for cancer patients, they are good advice to ask no matter what your condition. You should ask not only about what will happen to you, but also about the trial itself.

Don't be bamboozled or intimidated by a bunch of people in white coats with lots of letters after their names. It's your body, your health, and your time. They answer to you, or you don't sign on with them.

Your Checklist for Investigating Clinical Trials

About your participation in the study:

- ❏ What is the purpose of the study?
- ❏ What will the study do, and how will it do it?
- ❏ What is likely to happen to me if I don't participate in this study? If I do?
- ❏ Are there standard treatments that could benefit me? What are the advantages and disadvantages of these treatments compared with participating in this study?
- ❏ How could participating in the study affect my daily life?
- ❏ What side effects could I expect from the study? How do these compare with the side effects from standard treatments—or no treatment—and from the disease itself?
- ❏ How long will the study last? Will it require an extra time commitment from me?
- ❏ Will I have to spend time in the hospital? If so, how often and for how long?
- ❏ Will participating in the study cost me anything? (See also "Who Pays for What" in this chapter.)
- ❏ If I am harmed in the course of the study, what treatment would I receive? This information may be critical to getting your plan's approval to participate.
- ❏ What type of long-term follow-up care (after the study itself is over) is part of the study?

About the study itself:

- ❏ What is the purpose of the study? The people running it should be able to explain it in terms you can understand and evaluate.
- ❏ Who has reviewed and approved the study? People can't just experiment on human beings without subjecting the study plan to review. The review board may be in the hospital or medical school itself.
- ❏ Who is sponsoring the study? An outside sponsoring body—a government agency or foundation, for example—will usually subject the study to extensive review by outside experts in the field. If the hospital or medical school is sponsoring the study itself, there may be less review.
- ❏ How are the study data and patient safety being checked?
- ❏ Where will information from the study go? In a government-sponsored study, reports might go to the National Cancer Institute or the FDA.

Source: National Cancer Institute Website (see Appendix B).

Who Decides If You Are Eligible?

Both the people running the study and your health care plan will have a lot to say about whether you enroll in a clinical trial.

Talking to the White Coats

When you are faced with a serious condition, put all your energy into learning about, cooperating with, and succeeding in whatever standard therapies are available for your condition. Good doctors want you to be involved in making choices about your treatment, and you always have the right to turn down treatment. But don't forgo standard therapy and then place all your hope in untested treatments when your condition becomes more serious. If you pass up chemotherapy or radiation for an early-stage cancer because you fear it could be unpleasant or time consuming, for example, your options may be much more limited if your cancer returns or spreads.

If you are interested in participating in a clinical trial, check first with your own doctor or specialists. If there are facilities doing medical research in your area, the health section of your newspaper may contain advertisements soliciting people to participate in trials. The National Cancer Institute maintains a computer file about some 1,500 ongoing clinical trials. You can get this information from your doctor or by calling the Cancer Information Service (CIS) toll-free at 1-800-4-CANCER. A useful Website dealing with clinical trials is maintained by Centerwatch, Inc. (see Appendix B). Interest groups and support groups dealing with your condition can also help you find out what is available (see Appendix B).

If there is a clinical trial that could be suitable for you, you will first be evaluated by the study staff. They will be interested in your overall health, the progression of your disease, and your medical history, including your responses to any previous treatment you might have had. Research studies usually have strict requirements about who can be included. Whether or not you are accepted for a study might have nothing to do with your long-term prognosis. Indeed, you can be rejected for a clinical trial because you are not sick enough!

Your Personal Rx
Some doctors told us that patients can be pressured to participate in clinical trials. After all, important research can be jeopardized if patients won't participate, and current treatments were all once tested on trial participants. But don't let yourself be pressured into participating in a trial. If you have a serious illness, your energy should go into getting well, not into meeting someone else's needs.

You will also be asked to sign an informed consent form (more on this in Chapter 22). Even before you are evaluated for participation, the study itself should have passed muster with an institutional review board that includes medical, legal, and community representatives. Such review is required by federal law if public funds are used for the study. Many research facilities also use institutional ethics committees to provide advice about a person's continuation or termination in a clinical trial. If you want to know more, you can ask your doctor how to get in touch with these boards.

Talking to Your Plan

There have been a lot of reports of managed care plans denying their members permission to participate in a clinical trial for fear that the trial may cause side effects or complications that the plan would then be obliged to treat. Ask careful questions of your doctor, your plan, the people running the clinical trial, and perhaps your lawyer before proceeding.

Above all, don't do anything that would jeopardize either your health or your coverage. While it can be hard if you feel your life or that of a family member is at stake, use the same common sense you've been trained to use—since the age of 16—in a fender-bender. Don't sign anything, don't admit anything, and don't give up any rights until you have had a chance to get disinterested professional advice.

Off-Label Uses of Approved Drugs

After a drug is approved for one disease or condition, doctors can legally prescribe it for other conditions as well. Such a prescription is called an *off-label* use, because the manufacturer may not legally market the drug for any conditions that have not been approved. Off-label use is common in cancer treatment but occurs in the treatment of other conditions as well.

Some states have passed legislation requiring private insurers to cover off-label uses as long as published evidence and expert opinions on the value of the drugs in these uses is included in three major research compendia (collections). Medicare and Medicaid also cover off-label uses covered in these compendia. If your plan denies coverage for a prescription drug on the grounds that the prescribed use is off-label, check the law in your state, then see if you can appeal the plan's decision.

> **Healthspeak**
> An *off-label* use of a prescription drug is a use that has not been formally approved by the U.S. Food and Drug Administration. Doctors may legally prescribe off-label uses for approved drugs.

Investigational Procedures

Even if you are not being treated in a clinical trial, your plan or insurance company may decide that a procedure you want is investigational based on the rules we listed earlier. But it still may be covered.

Rules Can Be Overruled

Some plans simply provide exceptions to their own rules. One managed care plan, for example, throws away its own prohibitions on experimental and investigational treatments if:

Your Personal Rx

Some outside review panels reportedly *never* rule for the patient. You may do better bypassing the plan's review panel entirely and going directly to a specialist in your field who will take on your plan directly. But don't ever bypass your plan's precertification requirements, or your ability to recover your costs later could be threatened (see also Chapters 23 and 24).

➤ The patient can be expected to die within one year in the absence of effective treatment,

and

➤ Scientific data suggest that the treatment is promising.

Outside review of the treatment decision is common in such cases.

But expect the panel of medical professionals to be selected—and paid—by your plan. Who do you think they'll be working for?

If you have doubts that the panel will be impartial—or even informed—try to make sure that it includes specialists in treating your disease or condition. Amazingly enough, even in complex cases, you are not assured that, say, an oncologist (cancer specialist) will be involved in reviewing a request for a bone marrow transplant (used in treating some advanced cancers).

There Are Rules, and Then There Are Rules

While you have to abide by your plan's rules, *it* has to answer to a higher authority, and usually more than one (see Chapter 25 for more on this). Many of these authorities tell the plan what it must cover and thus override any other rules that may apply. For example, the Federal Employees Health Benefits Program (FEHBP) requires participating plans to cover high-dose chemotherapy with autologous bone marrow transplant (HDC/ABMT) for breast cancer that has spread to other places in the body, even though some studies have concluded that the benefits of this technique for this condition have not been proven.

Some states also require insurers to cover this procedure, but if your plan is self-insured (see Chapter 3), these laws would generally not apply. It's always worth checking the laws, as well as recent court decisions, in your state or region (see Chapters 24 and 25).

Who Pays for What?

Members of managed care plans sometimes face special problems and issues in deciding whether to participate in a clinical trial or obtain new, advanced treatments. You didn't ask to get sick, and you (or your employer) did have the foresight to get you health care coverage. You'll feel a lot better (trust us!) if you can get someone else to pay for your treatment.

Clinical Trials

If you are interested in participating in a clinical trial, one of your first questions should be about financial responsibility. Don't be embarrassed to ask the question! You may not find out about aid available to you unless you do.

Many clinical trials require only that the patient pay for transportation, parking, and lodging if travel away from home is required, and some may even cover those costs. But different institutions—as well as health care plans—have different arrangements and policies. If you or your plan are expected to cover some of the cost of participating in the trial, read your plan documents first. While managed care plans routinely exclude coverage for experimental or investigational treatments, some will cover such treatments in certain circumstances:

➤ You may want to ask if your health plan is part of a joint venture with research organizations and pharmaceutical companies or others to test the experimental treatment. If so, the plan may pay for the treatment even if it is more expensive than standard treatment.

➤ Some plans will cover drugs administered in clinical trials that have made it pretty far up the ladder to final approval, even if they have not been finally approved.

Next, talk to the people running the trial. Many institutions that undertake clinical trials have special staff people who spend all their time dealing with insurance companies and health care plans. They know how to make the case for the treatment you are planning to undergo in exactly the way your health care plan or insurance company will find convincing. Give them all the necessary information and see what they can do.

If, after taking these steps, you still can't get your treatment paid for, there may be financial aid available for you. Start with the hospital's social services office. If you are trying to get into a cancer-related trial, contact the National Institutes of Health (NIH) or the major interest and support groups (American Cancer Society and American Lung Association, for example) dealing with your condition.

House Call

When it comes to financing treatment at the frontiers of medicine, you may have to let others take the lead. The office staff at the bone marrow transplant clinic or clinical trial know more than you do about how the study can be "sold" to your plan or insurance company. They know the "special" words to use and those to avoid.

Investigational Treatments

If you or your doctor feel you would be a good candidate for a nonstandard or investigational treatment, you should start by reading your insurance policy or plan contract (if you don't have yours, read Chapter 3). If your policy or contract excludes coverage for experimental or investigational treatments, your doctor needs to submit documentation that the treatment falls within the boundaries of both standard medical practice and the terms of the contract. Vague terms in an insurance policy or health care coverage contract are supposed to be interpreted in favor of the policy holder.

If you do this and your plan needs further persuading, you may want to file a formal appeal (Chapter 23) or go to court (Chapter 24). Which route you choose should depend on your health status, how much time you have to make a treatment decision, and the chances that the plan will cooperate if asked nicely. Be guided by your doctor—and maybe your lawyer—not by your emotions.

The Least You Need to Know

➤ If you or a family member is diagnosed with a serious medical condition, put all your energy into cooperating with—and succeeding in—standard treatment.

➤ If standard treatment has not worked for you—or no standard treatment is available—you may want to consider participating in a clinical trial. A trial may give you access to a promising new treatment long before it is available to the general public. But the treatment could also turn out to be useless.

➤ You don't give up your rights as a patient just because you are taking part in a research study. You—and no one else!—should decide whether to participate in a clinical trial and whether to stop doing so. Check the informed consent form and ask the people running the clinical trial to clarify any questions you may have.

➤ While most plans don't cover experimental or investigational treatments, they often have exceptions to their own rules. Understand those exceptions before making treatment decisions.

➤ If an outside medical panel is convened to review your treatment request, keep an eye on its makeup. It's not uncommon for panels to lack specialists in the treatment being considered.

➤ If you have doubts about the review process, go directly to an expert in treating your condition. He or she is also likely to have experience in dealing with health plans and insurance companies.

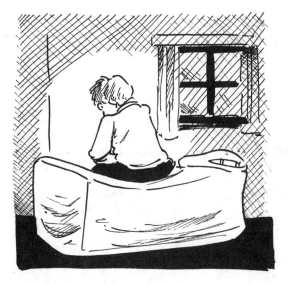

Chapter 19

Mental Health and Substance Abuse Treatment

In This Chapter

➤ How to get the help you need

➤ Your mental health professional

➤ What to expect of outpatient care

➤ What to expect of inpatient care

➤ Making the most of limited services

➤ When you have to take control

Do you or a loved one need help getting through difficult times? Maybe you are one of the many who suffer from depression or have a problem with alcohol. Perhaps your personal life is so stressful that you feel you need some counseling to help you get through the days. You checked your plan's booklet, and on one page it lists your mental health and substance abuse benefits. You're set, right?

Not necessarily.

Two obstacles could confront you:

➤ Your plan may be more restrictive in practice than on paper. In the worst case, you may get only a fraction of what you need and what you are entitled to. And your out-of-pocket costs may be higher than they are for other health care under your plan.

➤ Advocacy is key when you believe you are not getting the services you are promised by your managed care plan. But trying to be an advocate for yourself or a loved one at a time when you are least able (or energized) to be one can be almost impossible.

> ### House Call
>
> Fifty-two million Americans annually experience a mental health or substance abuse problem, but fewer than half ever seek treatment.

This chapter helps you evaluate your benefits and learn how to get what you need. We wrote this chapter for people with mental health or substance abuse problems. But it is also for the people who love them and might become responsible for their interactions with the health care system.

Finding Your Way to Help

First, determine what your plan provides; then find out what you have to do to get care.

What's in the Plan?

There is no single type of mental health plan. They vary widely. Some HMOs and other managed care plans enroll or hire mental health professionals directly. Others contract with specialty companies, called "carve-outs," whose only business is mental health (see Chapter 1 for more on carve-outs) or substance abuse treatment. Do not assume your care comes directly from your managed care company just because you have mental health coverage. Carve-out firms may have different phone numbers and addresses than your managed care plan, and often they have different rules for getting care. Some employers have employee assistance programs that may provide some short-term, problem-solving help to the employee. Expect to be seen by a clinical social worker, and don't expect long term psychotherapy.

Your Personal Rx

Many mental health problems are chronic conditions. You or a loved one may need specialty care or qualify for experimental treatment. Please look at Chapters 16, 17 and 18 which specifically cover these topics. They provide information that can be applicable to mental health treatment as well.

Their business can be nationwide, delivering mental health services to a variety of managed care plans around the country. They are sensitive to market demands, so they provide benefits that their purchasers, mainly employers or health plans, want. Competition among these firms is among the fiercest in the health care industry.

House Call

Mental health systems, as with all medical systems, are pushed to feed the hunger for data. Information systems are developed to collect and share outcomes data with employers and providers. This is where concerns for privacy can arise. See Chapter 22 for more information on keeping your health care records private.

Managed care mental health plans focus on which mental health professional will treat you; how many sessions the plan will pay for; whether inpatient care is required; what tests are needed; and what medicine is allowed.

Just like the treatment of other illnesses, the treatment of mental disorders and substance abuse problems is subject to the test of medical necessity. And the possibility (and fear) that under-treatment will result from the plan opting for the lowest-price treatment first exists in managed mental health services as it does in all of managed care.

Consumers who want some mental health services but who do not reach the diagnostic threshold for psychiatric disorders (for example, those responding to sources of stress, such as divorce or bereavement) may get a few sessions for evaluation purposes. They may not, however, be able to get referred to counseling as quickly as they would like. This is pretty hard to accept, especially when you look at your paycheck and see how much is deducted for health care premiums.

So if you need to evaluate a new plan, or are looking at your present plan for the first time, keep these questions in mind:

➤ Who are the mental health providers, and what are their qualifications?

➤ How do you get information on mental health providers? Be aware that printed lists are sometimes not available, and the only way you can get a provider is by giving the plan your zip code, whereupon they give you the names and some information on someone in your area.

➤ How many visits are offered by the plan? How many initial visits do you get before your mental health provider has to make a case for more care?

Your Personal Rx
One of the main complaints we heard from consumers and providers alike is the discrepancy between the number of visits the plan says it covers and the number of visits *you* are actually authorized. Be aware that these numbers may not match.

➤ How do you get an appointment? Do you call the plan, pick a psychiatrist or counselor, and schedule an appointment, or do you have to get a referral from your primary care doctor or pediatrician?

➤ Are you required to call a separate mental health plan telephone number and talk about your situation before being allowed to pick a provider?

➤ Is location important to you?

➤ Does the plan offer rehabilitation coverage? What about substance abuse (includes alcohol and drugs) detoxification?

➤ Does the plan have enough mental health providers so that waiting for an appointment is not an issue?

➤ How much are your copays and deductibles? In a PPO, a set copay may be $20 per visit, while an out-of-network therapist may be allowed 70 percent of his or her usual and customary charges, and you are left with the rest.

The Mental Health Parity Act, a federal law that goes into effect in 1998, bans annual and lifetime caps on mental healthcare benefits that are lower than caps established for physical care. Plans may, however, continue to specify different limits on inpatient treatment, different cost-sharing requirements, and different standards relating to medical necessity. Chemical and substance abuse treatments are excluded from these new parity requirements. The law will apply to employers with more than 50 employees.

Your Personal Rx

Whether you are choosing a plan, or about to use mental health care, always ask for a clear description of the plan's benefits and ask about complaint, grievance, and appeal procedures. You may have to act quickly, and it's best to know the steps.

If your present plan uses a carve-out firm and you change plans, your old carve-out plan may actually be part of your new plan. Check out who services mental health for your new plan and, if it is the same as your old plan, find out what you need to do to keep all your providers intact. Be advised that your actual benefits (number of visits, copays, and so on) may change.

If you are on medication, check out your drug coverage. Does it have a cap? If it does, flexible spending accounts (or your rainy day fund) can really come in handy (see Chapter 5 for more on this).

Getting Care

Managed care is based on gatekeepers, assessments, and rules. Mental health care is no different. You need to know which telephone numbers to call, if you need a referral and from whom, and where you can go for treatment. "There are many, many times during treatment when a treatment decision has to be made," one psychologist explained. "Each decision can involve therapists, doctors, and reviewers at a number of levels before the plan signs off on treatment."

Sometimes primary care doctors are involved. This can be iffy; they are not mental health specialists and may not recognize symptoms unless they are severe and highly characteristic of the disease. But managed care also relies on your contact and communication with primary care providers. Your physical symptoms may overlap with mental health concerns.

If your managed care plan requires you to get a referral from your primary care doctor, you will have to request it from her. If you have a child, you will have to get a referral from the pediatrician. We were told a number of times that "the sicker you are, the faster the referral," so don't be surprised if getting a referral and appointment take some time.

Make sure you understand the referral process, or you will add more stress to a stressful situation. The referral will allow a certain number of visits or a certain length of time during which the referral is valid. If you need more visits or your time runs out, you may have to come back to your primary doctor (most likely in concert with your therapist) and ask, even if your coverage says you can have 20 or even unlimited visits. If you need more visits in a calendar year than is allowed in the contract, your primary care doctor and therapist may have to make the case to the medical director of the plan.

Sometimes the therapist does not have to go back to the primary care doctor but can request more visits when he submits an outpatient treatment report (we are assuming the patient is being treated on an outpatient basis).

If you are in a plan that allows you to self-refer, that is, go to the therapist or counselor without the blessing of the primary care physician, you may be okayed for a certain number of visits. Self-referral doesn't mean you can go as long as you like or for the full number of visits allowed by your plan. The plan will review your therapist or counselor's treatment recommendation and either allow a set number of visits before another evaluation or suggest a new treatment path.

> **Your Personal Rx**
> If you have custody of a child but the child's health insurance is paid by the ex-spouse (or new spouse), make sure you have a copy of all documents, handbooks, and telephone numbers for the plan. If your child has to use the mental health benefits, you need these materials to understand what to do.

Your Mental Health Professional

Therapy is delivered in a one-on-one setting or in a small group. But behind those four walls is a surprising number of professionals, paraprofessionals, and clerical workers with jobs to do.

Who can deliver mental health and substance abuse care in a managed care setting? Your plan can include psychiatrists, psychologists, clinical social workers, psychiatric clinical nurse specialists, clinical social workers, marriage and family therapists, and licensed professional counselors. As in most of managed care, there is an emphasis on certification as a measure of the plan using quality professionals.

> **House Call**
>
> Psychiatric and substance abuse facilities and programs can include inpatient treatment, partial hospitalization, residential treatment, dual diagnosis units (for those with both alcohol and substance abuse problems), child and adolescent programs, geriatric programs, structured outpatient programs, halfway house/group home care, and intensive home-based services.

The therapist devises a treatment plan, and the plan must okay it or come up with something different. Who does this review? Physicians, psychologists, clinical social workers, and psychiatric clinical nurse specialists can conduct reviews at all points and certify (that is, say that the plan is in agreement with the therapist's decision) that the treatment is medically necessary.

But there have also been reports that clerical workers have done reviews. It is during the review that many people are denied care or therapy is limited more than they would like. Some complaints include referrals to counselors who lack requisite skill to handle more than a small part of treatment needs or too few authorized visits.

Your best ally may be your therapist. If you have one who is aggressive and willing to work his way up the line of reviewers, your chances of getting the treatment you both envision is better.

But keep in mind two things:

➤ Part of the move to guidelines and outcomes is the reliance by plans on a numerical formula that ranks severity of mental health problems. The plan uses the formula during the review process. If you don't have "the right numbers," you may get less treatment.

➤ There is concern among therapists that if he or she makes too many appeals on behalf of the patient to the plan, the therapist will be disenrolled—dropped from the plan.

Compare this with the referral sword that can hang over the heads of primary care physicians (see Chapter 11 for more on this), and you'll get an idea of how that pressure works.

When You Need Outpatient Care

Both mental health and substance abuse treatment are built on outpatient care. Where inpatient treatment would have been the choice a decade ago, outpatient treatment is now preferred. A number of years ago, there were reports about too many people fixed in the 30-day inpatient alcohol, drug, or mental health treatment regimes who didn't need to be there. The number of days of inpatient care seemed to match the insurance coverage.

Some outpatient care may be delivered by your primary care doctor. A little counseling from primary care doctors can help moderate drinking habits and improve overall health of problem drinkers, for example. One recent study found that a couple of 15-minute counseling sessions in the regular course of seeing patients, with a follow-up call a couple weeks after each session, reduced alcohol consumption. However, the type of health insurance and the physician specialty allowed to treat you will most likely influence the type of treatment you get.

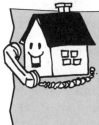

House Call

Chances are that if you are depressed and see a psychiatrist or psychologist, you will probably receive psychotherapy and/or antidepressant medication. Primary care doctors or master's level therapists in group settings are more likely to give you more advice-oriented counseling.

What exactly happens between your therapist or counselor and the plan? The managed care plan will tell your therapist that you are authorized for a certain number of visits that should be completed by a particular date. This may not be your allotment of visits available in your health plan booklet; it is the number of visits initially decided by the plan for you.

If your therapist thinks you need more visits, he or she will need to complete a Patient Evaluation and Treatment plan before the last authorized visit or before a certain date. He then must supply a clinical update if additional visits are required, and another decision must be made.

When You Need Inpatient Care

Nowhere is the tension between mental health treatment and managed care more striking than in decisions over inpatient services. For the therapist, hospitalization may mean a place for treatment or part of the treatment itself, while the managed care plan may see it as a failure of outpatient therapy. The therapist or family may believe that the hospital is the place to protect the patient, and the managed care company may counter with "Have you tried outpatient or community supports?" Hospitalization may also provide a chance for consultation or testing that may not be possible in outpatient care, especially if the diagnosis is complex. Further testing may be necessary to find out what is contributing to the symptoms and may lead to changes in treatment and medications.

If you or a loved one needs inpatient care, be prepared for a very short visit. Utilization review may approve inpatient psychiatric treatment but may authorize a much smaller number of days than requested. Sometimes alcohol and drug dependence diagnoses are even more restricted, limiting inpatient care to detoxification.

As you can see, there are a lot of pushes and pulls.

If you and the therapist feel that inpatient care is absolutely necessary, your therapist will have to be able to fight for you, especially for increasing days in inpatient care. He will have to get permission at every step. The outpatient therapist and inpatient therapist may be different people.

If this is what you want and need, be prepared to be—or have—an advocate. The advocate may be the therapist, but if you are not able to work with the therapist in dealing with your plan, try to enlist a spouse, parent, or other family member.

Keep on top of discharge plans. Some therapists have only inpatient practices and may be at odds with the outpatient therapist over treatment and discharge plans. If you are unhappy with the treatment or information you are getting, enlist your outpatient therapist to get the information you need for a clear picture so that any conflict can reach the resolution you need.

After you are discharged, keep your follow-up appointments—or demand them if none are scheduled. If you'd had surgery, nobody would have to remind you to have the stitches taken out. Think of post-hospital mental health care in the same way.

House Call

Day treatment has become a popular substitute for longer inpatient treatment. It may run most of the day, and placement may be for a number of months.

What happens when there are mental health problems along with physical problems, as is often the case with substance abuse? Are both sides aware of the other treatment? This should be the norm in an HMO, but, with carve-outs, you should monitor information exchanges between mental health and physical care providers. In a PPO, that conduit among your doctors may be you.

Pay attention to making sure everyone treating you knows about what else is going on. Sometimes the alliance among doctors who treat both body and mind is the key to getting the right treatment for you.

If Your Plan Has Limited Services

Some mental health benefits are more generous than others. If you change plans, continuity in your care may be a major problem.

Talk to your therapist and see what can be accomplished within the limits of your system, where problems may occur as you go through treatment, and what you might be able to do to make the best use of your plan within its limits.

Good managed care companies can put together good case management teams that can make the most of the benefits offered across the health plan. See if the therapist is setting objectives for treatment with the patient/family within the limits of the benefits package and plan for what happens when those benefits run out.

Managed care companies often limit the drugs that can be prescribed to their approved list (see Chapter 16 for more on this). Check on the status of therapeutic substitutions and whether they are equivalent to your present drug regime.

House Call

Managed care plans typically limit prescribing drugs to those indications approved by the FDA. For instance, some drugs approved for the treatment of convulsions could be used for the treatment of bipolar (manic-depressive) disorder. This is called an off-label use and may be unreimbursed or require special appeals in many plans. For more on off-label uses of drugs, see Chapter 18.

In psychotherapy, the therapeutic relationship between the patient and therapist is important to the patient's recovery. However, there may be times when you have to change plans and your therapist is not part of the new plan. You may have to pay out of pocket to continue that relationship. Check to see if you can negotiate on the fee. Your therapist may be willing to do this to keep the therapeutic relationship going. If you have a flexible spending account or have heeded our advice in Chapter 5 to establish a rainy day fund, that money may be useful here. If you must change therapists, go over the list with your current therapist for a recommendation.

How to Be an Advocate

The most common complaints received by the American Psychiatric Association's managed care hot line were:

➤ Denial of care for long-accepted disorders

➤ Excessive demands for sensitive patient data

➤ Untrained clerks following rigid rules in denying treatment

➤ Deceptive advertising of benefits by plans

➤ Interruption of treatment

The Institute of Medicine, an agency chartered by Congress to supply studies to the federal government, recently recommended better protections for those enrolled in managed behavioral health plans. Until these protections are adopted, what can you do to protect yourself and your loved ones?

➤ Ask why this course of treatment is the best course of treatment for this person. Ask the same question if and when there are changes in treatment or medication. Take notes.

➤ If you or your loved one has a chronic mental health or substance abuse condition, be vigilant. You will have to stay on top of treatment developments as you would for any other chronic disease (see Chapter 16).

➤ You will also have to stay on top of the type of mental health practitioner who should be treating the patient. Can a social worker do the job? Is a psychiatrist really necessary? What about a pharmapsychotherapist? Because those with Ph.D.s or M.S.W.s (Master of Social Work) charge lower prices than medical doctors (psychiatrists and the variations thereof), some managed care mental health plans push patients toward non-M.D. practitioners, sometimes at the expense of quality of treatment. But Ph.Ds and M.S.W.s also provide quality services. Essentially, you have to make sure whoever treats you or a loved one has the right qualifications. This is also where your advocacy skills can really be tested.

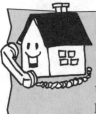

House Call

Maintaining privacy is often of particular concern to those undergoing mental health treatment. This is especially true of those receiving treatment in a managed health care setting because of the number of people involved in decisions and reviews (more on privacy in Chapter 22).

➤ Pay special attention to the elderly. Psychotic behavior, depression, or memory loss are not always part of the aging process. Mental health problems among the elderly often go undiagnosed because they don't ask or communicate well. Elderly patients may be particularly unsuited to the negotiating for care that can go on in managed mental health plans because they often believe there is a stigma to mental illness and because they are used to traditional, or fee-for-service, medicine.

➤ Find out what to do in a psychiatric emergency: how your plan defines it, how your therapist or counselor defines it, and where to meet between the two. If you or your loved one is on a new medication, make sure you understand what the side effects may be and what an adverse reaction may entail. If either of the above occurs, make sure you understand what you need to do. Is it an emergency or merely urgent (see Chapter 14 on understanding the difference between the two)? Whom do you contact, and where do you go for treatment?

➤ Ask how the doctors are paid. Information that plans are required to share with you can include how providers are paid. Some courts have said that a patient must know whether his or her medical advice is influenced by self-serving financial considerations created by the health insurance provider.

➤ Always get a copy of your records and, in particular, your diagnosis. If you feel there is a delay in treatment, inadequate treatment, or no follow-up care, and you want to do some research on what you should be receiving, you need your diagnosis as a baseline.

➤ Check out your local support groups and family support groups. You may want to contact your local chapter of the Alliance for the Mentally Ill. They have support groups, know the status of state law, and have good information and reading lists.

➤ It can be difficult to find out what standards mental health plans use for making care decisions. This is often considered part of their proprietary "business" information. However, as competition heats up, and employers ask about it, some are willing to offer information.

➤ And finally, don't underestimate the stress mental illness or substance abuse can bring to the entire family. Find out if the managed care plan has family support services. Watch the effects on your own health if you are a primary caretaker for a person with psychiatric problems.

The Least You Need to Know

➤ Know the benefits to which you are entitled. If your plan uses a specialty firm for mental health and substance abuse services (a carve-out), know the phone numbers, addresses, and rules for using those services. They can be different from the rest of your managed care plan.

➤ What you see is not necessarily what you get. Your plan document may say that you are entitled to a maximum of 20 visits, but your plan may pay for only ten, based on its assessment of what you need.

➤ Managed mental health and substance abuse treatment require that the medical necessity test be met just as in the treatment of any other illness. Your therapist may have to be your advocate when the plan reviews the amount and type of treatment you get.

➤ If you can't do it, get someone to be your advocate and make sure you get the treatment you need.

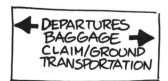

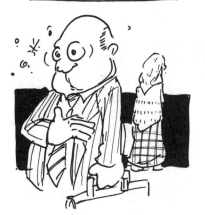

Chapter 20

When You're Out of Town

In This Chapter

➤ Getting care on a business trip

➤ Solving health problems on vacation

➤ Overseas travel and managed care

➤ College kids and health care

Summer. The drive, the scenery, that sunset. Then again, it can be the flu, the fracture, the malaria.

What do you do when you're not at home, and home means your health plan's *service area*? Where do you get care when your town is Minneapolis, but you're on business in Seattle? Buenos Aires is not currently in your service area, so what do you do for health care there? Can your newly minted Ivy Leaguer continue her coverage under your Chicago health plan?

This chapter covers what you need to know when you, or members of your family, hit the road.

Your Personal Rx

Your plan's service area specifically affects HMO members. HMOs have geographic areas in which they deliver services. You are usually restricted to receiving your care within the service area, unless it is an emergency or urgent. If you move out of your service area, you may no longer be covered by your plan.

Healthspeak

Reciprocal agreements are agreements among certain HMOs that allow members to use other HMO facilities and networks while traveling, and diagnosis and treatment of a condition cannot be delayed until you return to the plan's service area. Sometimes this is limited to emergency care only. Often members of the American Association of Health Plans, a national trade association for HMOs, maintain reciprocity agreements.

Take One Business Trip, Add Strep Throat

You aren't the first to wake up at 4 a.m. with a raging sore throat, three states west of home. Even the best sales managers can be felled by microbes.

What do you do first: Call the front desk and ask for the nearest doctor or hospital, or call your health plan? We suggest the health plan.

If you are a member of an HMO, it may have a *reciprocal agreement* with other HMOs near your hotel where you can receive urgent or emergency care.

If there are no reciprocal agreements, your urgent care line may be able to recommend a physician in the area.

If you are on your own, ask the hotel's front desk. When you go to the doctor (or hospital), be sure to take your ID card with you and submit your claims immediately. Even when you are in prepaid health care, you occasionally have to pay up front. In those situations, people often forget to submit their bills or submit them months later, just as they did when they had fee-for-service insurance.

Also check with your plan if you have a temporary assignment or sabbatical outside your service area. For instance, if you need to be on site in Houston for six weeks but your health plan is in Mobile, get guidance from your plan for health care. Some plans specifically state what is covered if you temporarily reside outside the service area, while others address it under the general procedures for out-of-area care.

Saving Your Vacation

Let's see, you've stopped the newspaper, your neighbor's son will feed the cats, and the airline tickets are in your right...no, left pocket. Are you forgetting anything?

Check your wallet and make sure you have everyone's plan ID cards. You always take your credit cards and driver's license, and these can be just as important.

No one likes to think about it, but everything from insect bites to heart attacks can ruin a vacation. If you talk to five people, you will get five horror stories about a trip-turned-medical-nightmare.

Take a few minutes and follow our travel checklist:

➤ Pack that ID card.

➤ Pack your member handbook for quick reference. This should include the urgent care number.

➤ If you are a member of an HMO, check to see if your plan has a reciprocity agreement with a plan near your destination. A reciprocity agreement covers you for medically necessary outpatient services (except prescription drugs) when provided by a participating HMO.

➤ Pack the prescription medicine you may need. Make sure you have enough and don't run out mid-trip. If you need a refill, make sure you get it before the trip. Refills and prescriptions may not be covered beyond your plan's participating pharmacies. If necessary, call your pharmacy and ask for a month's supply with approval by your doctor. Medications for travel-related problems, such as motion sickness, may not be covered.

➤ Pack the telephone numbers of your doctors and dentists (and their office hours).

When you are in a managed care plan, getting health care while you are far away is very similar to getting medical care when you are at home. Distance is of no consequence. Know what your policy contains and when you need a referral. Follow the steps you need for referral as you do when you are home. If you have an ear infection, still call your primary care physician to get the referral process going. Your plan's urgent care line, may be able to find a doctor in the area.

If you are under care, let your doctor know you are going to be away and the dates, so that an out-of-town call will be answered promptly. Make sure you review your plan handbook to see if there are limitations on out-of-town care.

Most often, late term pregnancies, the terminally ill, or patients with medically unstable conditions need the medical director's approval before leaving. One person with a chronic liver disease made arrangements through her doctor for a contact in the country she was visiting, just in case she needed medical care. Her doctor at home had trained the European doctor.

Be sure to submit any claims immediately. If you wait too long, your plan may not cover your out-of-town care, and you will be left holding the bill.

> **Your Personal Rx**
> If you are in a Medicare HMO, check the plan. If you live out of the area 90 days or more, you may lose your coverage, or your plan may allow nonemergency or non-urgent care outside the service area only up to a specific amount per calendar year. Medicare noncovered expenses, such as hospital inpatient deductibles, are your responsibility.

And schedule your follow-up care at home. Often, follow-up care is not covered for out-of-town services, unless you get permission from the medical director.

Emergency Visits

The keys to emergency care away from home are the same as emergency care at home: Notify the plan that you need care, take your health plan cards with you, and notify the plan about any hospitalizations within 24 hours. Call 911 (or its equivalent) when necessary. Distance doesn't change the steps (see Chapter 14 for more on emergency care).

People run to the emergency room quicker on vacation, especially if the local doctors are overloaded and can't fit you in as quickly as you need. Ask about urgent care or walk-in clinics. You can often find them in vacation areas. Still, call your doctor or plan and let them know where you are going and why, and take your information with you.

You may also have to call the plan to get claims information for your vacation ER visit. Sometimes ID cards don't have the address of where to send claims. You may be able to call collect for out-of-area emergencies if you don't have a toll-free number for your plan. When people don't have their information on hand, hospitals often ask them to call patient accounts to finish off the necessary paperwork.

Your Personal Rx
Be sure to call the plan named on your medical card. If your insurer has lots of different plans, don't call their main number; take the time to find the right number. The company may have hundreds of different plans in different states and the people at the main number may not give you the right information.

Be prepared to pay your copays and deductibles. The obligation to pay copays does not expire when you leave town. They apply even to out-of-town emergencies.

What if you need hospitalization? If you don't notify the plan, usually within 24 hours of admission to a hospital, you run the risk of the plan not reimbursing you. If you need more than overnight hospital care, you may be moved to a local plan hospital as soon as your medical condition permits. This is usually coordinated through utilization review. Make sure you or someone else keeps up communication with you plan throughout the episode.

If you visit the ER on vacation, even if it wasn't on your itinerary, take a little phone time to get everything straight. If you do, you'll have a lot less to deal with after you get home, and you can keep that "vacation glow" a little longer.

We know you want to clear your head and enjoy the time off, so if we can boil this part down to one rule, this is it. If you don't get and convey all the information to the hospital and to your plan, you may be the monkey in the middle. Then you have to pay first and ask questions later.

A P.S. for the vacation athletes: Take a first-aid book along. We won't divulge any more family lore. Let's just say it had to do with Thanksgiving, a football, and a very large nephew. Someone may need to stabilize the injury on the way to the hospital. And someone should grab the "star's" wallet with the health card and the phone numbers.

Dental Emergencies

Why is it that rock candy in Maine can set off a dental emergency? Or your kids collide during flashlight tag at Grandma's, sending a front tooth flying? If you are out of town, your dental plan may be provide a certain amount of money for stabilizing your condition, and that's it. All further dental work would have to be done by your regular dentist or dental specialist on the plan list for the plan to cover your costs.

You may also have to pay the full bill for the out-of-town dentist and then submit a claim. Remember, sometimes your dental benefits are provided by a "carve-out" plan, and you need to use a different telephone number and address to ask questions or submit claims.

Kids Away from Home

If your neighbor offers to take your daughter along to the beach so that her daughter will have a good time, don't forget to send a few pieces of information. Give your neighbor your plan information, including urgent care numbers and plan identification numbers, along with a permission slip for emergency medical care. Also supply her with any information on allergies and other medical conditions that may crop up.

If your children visit relatives, provide the same type of information. Plan information is not genetically conveyed. Even Grandpa needs to know who should be contacted and some of the basic rules required by your managed care plan for care away from home.

International Travel

We know that foreign travel immediately conjures up images of exotic places, food, and—shots. If you are going overseas and need immunizations, advance planning is necessary. Some immunizations need to be given weeks before you go, or a series of shots may be needed.

Your plan may only cover routine immunizations as part of its preventive health program. Check to see what shots it offers for overseas travel, where to get them, and what you have to pay.

The biggest risks to travelers abroad are intestinal illnesses, motor vehicle accidents, and malaria. There are medical evacuation services for the serious illnesses. American embassies have lists of English-speaking doctors and dentists who generally have had some training in the U.S.

> **Your Personal Rx**
> Check with your plan before you leave the country. Many plans have travel advisory services. Their travel nurse gives information on immunizations; medications to bring along for travel-related illnesses; food, water, and insect precautions; and so on. Your plan may be able to provide you with some useful information for your upcoming trip.

If you are hospitalized abroad, have someone call your plan for assistance. There are still charges for health care, and arrangements for payment must be made. You will need to schedule follow-up care as well, so arrange to have any records transferred back to your primary care physician.

Your College Student

As the college staff patiently answered questions about dorm food, activity fees, and bike thefts, a murmur swept through the audience as they noticed the next order of business: health care. "What exactly does student health services provide? Do they give allergy shots? Can I keep her on my health insurance, or should I get the college insurance?"

One parent rose from the audience and pleaded with her fellow parents. "I am a nurse in a doctor's office near a university. Please, please make sure your student knows about his or her health plan. I am tired of being yelled at by parents, health plans, and carping students all because they didn't even know what plan they had. Some discovered at our office that they weren't covered by their parent's plan."

You and your student have conquered the complexities of SATs, applications, and student aid. You can also figure out a health plan for them.

Your Personal Rx
Most colleges and universities have mandatory health fees to pay for student health center services. Some states allow a waiver of those fees if the student submits proof of their private health care coverage.

If your student stays within your plan's service area, his or her coverage can usually continue under your plan. Some plans require certification that your child is a full-time student. Some plans insure children up to age 19, and then you must show that they are attending school. If your student stays in the service area, the only change they need to make is possibly moving from a pediatrician to an internist or family practitioner for primary care.

If you are in an HMO, your policy may, in effect, cover only urgent or emergency care away from home, and prescription drugs may not be covered unless your student gets them back home. Essentially, your student is treated as though she is traveling out of town. If you are in an HMO that is statewide, however, you may be able to get all her care, including routine care, at the plan's facilities or network in Collegetown.

If you are in a PPO, the same types of rules apply. Medical care she receives may be out-of-network, with the required coinsurance and physician payments dictated by out-of-network procedures.

You are probably used to working from lists for applications, recommendations, and packing. Here's a list to help you unravel yet another complicated consequence of higher education:

➤ Verify your child's coverage before he goes to college. You may need to certify that he is a full-time student, usually through the registrar. A graduate student may not be covered under your policy and may need to buy one on his own.

➤ If you choose to enroll your student in the insurance plan offered through the college, check to see if it covers your student when he is away from school. Some policies run from August to August, so that students are covered during the summer. Sometimes summer coverage is extra.

Your Personal Rx
Watch out for caps on major medical coverage offered through the college. Student coverage is much more of a "bare bones" policy than those offered by employers. It has to be affordable to someone attending college.

➤ Ask what services are covered through the health fees paid to the college. If, combined with emergency care from your managed care plan, it provides the care your student needs, you're set. If it doesn't, you may want to buy the college insurance plan. If you do, you will have to alert your health plan. You will have to fill out forms for coordination of benefits (see Chapter 5) the same way you may have to do for a spouse.

➤ If your student pares down to part-time status, she may put her coverage under your plan at peril. If your child drops out of school, even for a semester, she may be dropped from your coverage and may not be able to get coverage under your plan again if she goes back. Check out under what circumstances your student remains covered under your plan.

➤ If your student drops your coverage for the college policy and then wants back on your plan, it may not work. Students are not necessarily able to get back on their parent's policies after they drop the coverage.

➤ If you buy a student plan and your student drops a semester with intentions to go back, find out if you can buy extended coverage during that time. As with most policies, when a student leaves college, he leaves the policy. If he takes a semester off, get a short-term medical policy; they are available.

What happens when she gets that diploma? If your student was covered under your family plan, she may be able to get a temporary continuation under COBRA (see Chapter 7 for more on this). Next stop, employer-sponsored health care coverage!

The Least You Need to Know

➤ When you travel, take your health plan ID card along with your driver's license and credit cards. If you are away on business or pleasure, that ID gives you access to medical care.

➤ Wherever you are, at home or abroad, get in touch with your managed care plan whenever you need medical care. You may need approval, and you could probably use some guidance. If you don't get in touch, it may cost you more than your vacation budget.

➤ If you are going overseas, your plan may not cover all the immunizations you need. Allow enough time to get all the shots you need.

➤ Check, and double-check, your student's coverage on your plan. If you need more coverage, look into the optional college plan. Whatever you choose, take time to prepare him or her on how to use what they have and to carry their health care card along with their student ID.

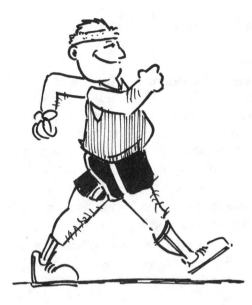

Chapter 21

Stepping Up to Bat: The Rest of Your Health Care Team

In This Chapter

➤ Moving beyond traditional medicine

➤ Will your plan pay for alternative clinicians?

➤ And something extra: classes, discounts, and support groups brought to you by your health plan

If your idea of health care is a shot, a prescription, or surgery—or your idea of a doctor is limited to people with M.D. or D.O. after their name—it's time for an update. Here are a few facts for you to digest:

➤ Washington state has passed legislation requiring all managed care plans and insurers to make alternative health care available to subscribers.

➤ A large, northwestern insurer offers members a chance to buy a prepaid electronic card they can use to pay for discounted services from participating providers offering acupuncture, massage, physical therapy, herbal remedies, nutritional supplements, and other products.

➤ A large, northeastern HMO offers access to alternative health care providers to over a million members.

Healthspeak
Complementary and *alternative* medicine covers a broad range of healing philosophies, approaches, and therapies. They can be used alone (often referred to as *alternative*), in combination, or in addition to conventional therapies (sometimes known as *complementary*). They are not taught widely in U.S. medical schools, nor are they generally available in hospitals. For information about complementary and alternative medicine and research, contact the Office of Alternative Medicine at the National Institutes of Medicine (see the tearout card).

➤ Mind-body medicine, which deals with how your mind can affect your health, is one of the hottest fields in medicine.

➤ The federal Agency for Health Care Policy and Research (AHCPR), a government research arm for developing standards of appropriate care, has found that spinal manipulation, often performed by chiropractors and osteopaths (see Chapter 2 for more on these), is safe and effective for certain patients with lower back pain.

➤ You may be able to choose acupuncture as a form of anesthesia for your next surgery.

➤ Your health plan may offer you stress-reduction classes, mall walks with your medicines, and child care referrals for working parents after childbirth.

No, you haven't wandered into some tie-dyed, new-age wonderland. And this chapter is *not* about turning away from mainstream medicine. It's about the way many plans are integrating mainstream medicine with areas of medicine that once were considered unconventional but are now being considered *complementary*. It's also about the way your plan may be working to support you in maintaining a healthy lifestyle. This chapter is about expanding your health care choices—and your managed care plan's role in these choices.

You Say "Doctor," I Say "Alternative Clinician"

A *clinician* is someone who sees, evaluates, and treats patients. As we have discussed in previous chapters, clinicians you will see in a managed care plan can include lots of people. Some, such as advanced practice nurses and physician assistants, usually work with physicians and under their supervision. Others practice in areas that overlap with the scope of traditional physicians' medical practice: psychologists, podiatrists, and optometrists, to name a few.

In this chapter, we want to talk about a third group, once considered unorthodox at best, now increasingly part of mainstream, traditional medicine. These are nonphysician clinicians, though some plans may consider them physicians for definitional purposes (that means they are willing to pay for their services). Three types of nonphysician clinicians are licensed and regulated by many states: chiropractors, practitioners of Oriental medicine and acupuncture, and naturopaths. Some states also license massage therapists and homeopathic practitioners.

If your managed care plan pays for services by alternative clinicians, it may not pay for their services under certain circumstances. For example, your plan may pay for massage as a component of physical therapy, but not for other health problems. So if you need massage therapy during your recovery from a knee injury, it may be part of your plan's covered services for physical therapy, but if you want to use massage to deal with migraines, your plan may not pay.

One of the reasons coverage for alternative medicine is limited is the scarcity of scientific journals, studies, and evidence supporting it. Traditional medicine is steeped in hard science validation. Managed care, with its emphasis on guidelines and outcomes based on this type of evidence, may decide that only a few conditions are eligible for treatment under the plan. The full range of treatments an alternative clinician can do may not "fit the code" for utilization review.

Your Personal Rx

If you want to consult a medical practitioner in a field that your state does not license and regulate, check to see if the person has graduated from an accredited institution of professional training and has obtained certification from an appropriate professional association.

However, consumer demand, more state regulation, and more data on alternative treatments are leading to change in making alternative medicine part of managed care plans. Observers expect the number of clinicians and benefits to grow dramatically in the future.

House Call

The cost of alternative medicine is no small change. A 1993 landmark study estimated that 60 million Americans used alternative medical therapies at an estimated cost of $13.7 billion. Annual visits to alternative providers exceeded the number of visits to all U.S. primary care doctors. One-third of all alternative therapy seems to be associated with health promotion and disease prevention.

But Americans tend to keep their doctors in the dark about their "other" medical care. Seventy percent of patients who said they used alternative therapies never mentioned it to their physicians.

Let's just say communication on both the patient's and provider's end has been lax. We've stressed communication all the way along, so tell your doctor or specialist if you are using alternative medicines and therapies. Tell your alternative clinician about your physician care and medications. There is always a chance that, unless you coordinate the information, everyone will be working at cross purposes. This could be dangerous, especially in terms of drug interactions. And if you need emergency care, you want your primary care doctor to be familiar with your treatments.

Your Personal Rx
If you have to call your plan's urgent care line with questions about whether you or a loved one needs urgent or emergency care, be sure to tell them if you are using any alternative treatments, including dietary supplements. They can't assess the situation without all the information.

The list of questions you ask your alternative clinician are very similar to those you ask any doctor:

➤ Have you treated other patients like me (with similar symptoms, the same age, the same gender, and so on)?

➤ What are the expected results?

➤ Of what does the treatment(s) consist and how often will it be necessary?

➤ What are the advantages and disadvantages, the risks, and possible side effects?

➤ When will I know if the treatment is beneficial?

Ask that your alternative clinician communicate any diagnosis, therapeutic plans, and follow-up treatments with your primary care doctor or specialist. If they are in conflict over treatment, get the full story from both to *your* satisfaction.

Chiropractors

Chiropractic is the oldest of the alternative clinical professions (in the U.S., that is) and is the most widely licensed. Licensure is available in all 50 states and the District of Columbia. Many chiropractors practice alone in the same way that much of the medical profession has always done, but others practice as part of chiropractic group or interdisciplinary provider group.

Some of the problems chiropractors routinely treat include:

➤ Lower back pain

➤ Problems with the neck and upper back

➤ Headaches

➤ Visceral disorders

Chiropractors (also known as doctors of chiropractic, or D.C.s) and osteopaths (also known as doctors of osteopathy, or D.O.s) may often address spinal and related problems in similar ways, including spinal manipulation. (For more on osteopaths, see Chapter 2.) Like D.O.s and M.D.s, but unlike physical therapists, D.C.s can also diagnose patient problems and address problems with the nervous system. Both D.C.s and D.O.s may approach patient care from a wide range of disciplinary and professional perspectives, so ask a lot of questions about your likely treatment, care, and prognosis. And, as you would with any medical practitioner, look at qualifications, personal referrals from friends and family, and personal "fit" in choosing a practitioner.

In the past, chiropractors and practitioners of traditional medicine have not worked well together, and many traditional doctors discouraged patients from consulting chiropractors. Today, however, the AHCPR has placed its seal of approval on chiropractic treatment for some musculoskeletal conditions. As a result, some chiropractors believe that medical prudence could require doctors to refer patients for chiropractic treatment before recommending back surgery.

If you are in a managed care plan, your ability to consult a chiropractor could vary widely. If you are in a network plan with no gatekeeper, you may have access to both in-network and out-of-network providers. Read your plan's Summary Plan Description (see Chapter 3 for more of this) and provider directory to find out about your options.

If you are in a tightly managed plan such as a staff- or group-model HMO, or if you depend on your primary care doctor to outline your treatment options, you may have access to a chiropractor within the plan—or you may never hear about chiropractic care. Your treatment options may depend on your doctor's individual perspective and experience, as well as on your own health status. So if you believe you could benefit from chiropractic care—and especially if your doctor has recommended back surgery—take the initiative yourself. Talk to your plan and ask your chiropractor to do so, too. Your back and your pocket book may thank you!

Oriental Medicine and Acupuncture

Acupuncture is an ancient medical technique that relies on piercing parts of the body with needles to treat disease or relieve pain. Practitioners of Oriental medicine and acupuncture are licensed in 24 states and the District of Columbia. Three states offer licensure for specialists practicing under the supervision of a physician. Unlike chiropractors, practitioners of acupuncture and Oriental medicine are not typically permitted to use the title "doctor" or "physician."

Managed care plans differ widely in their provision of benefits for acupuncture therapy. Some plans cover it if the treatment is medically necessary and delivered within the scope of the acupuncturist's license. Other plans may limit coverage for acupuncture to its use as a form of anesthesia when performed by a covered health care provider in connection with surgery covered under the plan.

If you are interested in acupuncture therapy, get a copy of your plan's SPD and read the rules. Then, be prepared to offer evidence that the treatment is medically necessary and appropriate.

Naturopathy

Do you hate drugs, knives, and needles? Naturopathy may be for you. It's a system of treating diseases that relies largely on natural agencies such as air, water, and sunshine and rejects the use of drugs and medicines. While naturopaths (doctors of naturopathy, or N.D.s) are licensed in only some states, they practice in a number of states with no licensure laws. Some may practice under the supervision of a physician, others independently.

233

Your ability to get coverage for naturopathic treatments could depend on state law, on whether your plan is self-insured by an employer, and on the practitioner's practice arrangement. Some states require insurance companies licensed to do business within their borders to cover certain treatments and practitioners. Find out the law in your state by calling the state insurance commissioner's office listed in your local phone book.

But even if naturopathy is covered in your state, your *plan* may not have to cover it if the plan is self-insured (see Chapter 3 for a definition of self-insurance). Your employer's human resources office should be able to tell you whether the plan is self-insured or insured through an insurance company if you can't figure it out from your plan documents.

Your ability to be reimbursed for treatments could also depend on whether the N.D. practices in conjunction with an M.D. or D.O. If the treatments are prescribed by a traditional doctor and delivered by the N.D., your chances of reimbursement may be greater.

And Complements of Your Health Plan

Your managed care plan doesn't want you to get sick (and cost it money). So many plans make it easy for you to make good health a part of your lifestyle. And those extras the plan offers can pay off for you in time, money, and good health. Here are some of the extras you can expect from your plan:

➤ Health newsletters that keep you up-to-date with new developments and jog your memory on good health habits and preventive care

➤ Telephone-based advice services (see also Chapter 11)

➤ Self-care books dealing with preventive care and advice on when to seek medical treatment

➤ Health-risk appraisals that can point out health-destructive behaviors you may not even be aware of

HMOs are particularly adept at patient counseling and education programs that are especially effective if you are dealing with a chronic health condition (see Chapter 16). Some of these programs include asthma, cholesterol, diabetes management, and anti-stress and relaxation techniques.

You may need a referral from your doctor for programs like cholesterol or diabetes education. Then again, you can take a proactive approach and ask them for a referral before they ask you.

New member of the family arriving soon? No, we're not talking about your daughter's gerbil (or your mother-in-law); we're talking about a new baby. Your plan probably offers special prenatal or maternity education programs or materials (learn how to care for your little bundle of joy *before* she arrives!).

Some plans also offer new parent support groups and special pediatric CPR courses.

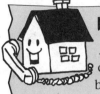

House Call

As far as we know, no HMO offers toy clean-up at 9 p.m. or grocery delivery services for new parents. Next time you pass their suggestion box...

What about the senior members? With the increase in Medicare enrollees in managed care plans, more programs are serving those over 65. HMOs are offering geriatric assessments, care management programs, nutrition, health lectures on aging, and the mall walks that keep you out and about.

Activities that may be offered directly by your employer or your health plan, often for free, include:

➤ Exercise and fitness programs, nutrition education, smoking cessation programs, and weight and stress management activities, including movement programs for overweight kids. Yoga and meditation may also be available through your health plan.

➤ Health incentives that allow you to receive cash or lower health care premiums with proof that you have quit smoking, lost weight, or participate in wellness programs.

➤ Education and training programs that can put you in charge of your own health, including managing your child's asthma or your lower-back pain and coping with grief or serious illness.

Other time and money savers? Many plans have teamed up with health clubs to offer discounts on memberships or to waive initiation fees. HMOs have even negotiated discounts for sport and workout equipment for their members with participating sporting goods stores. Some offer discounts to participating massage therapists. And if you clip recipes, don't throw away your plan newsletter. Low fat, vegetarian, and other healthy recipes may be listed next to the article on using emergency services.

Many plans also provide links to good childcare, a valuable commodity. They can help find child care centers convenient to your home or work and sometimes negotiate discounts at participating centers. These centers usually meet certain child care standards.

If you've suffered through a serious illness, ask your plan about its support groups. A sampling of support groups for cancer patients offered by a regional HMO include patients with any cancer diagnosis; women with newly diagnosed breast cancer; post-treatment breast cancer survivors; gynecological cancer; bone marrow transplant candidates and patients; patients with a brain tumor; and prostate cancer patients.

The programs may sometimes be hard to get to, and it's often hard to find the time to go. Check out if your plans have brown bag lunches. Heck, everybody has to eat sometime. Remember, you already paid for these freebies when you paid your health care premium.

The Least You Need to Know

➤ Check to see if your plan offers chiropractic services. Your chances are pretty good that it's on the list.

➤ If you are interested in alternative therapies, ask if your plan offers the type you want. If it does, the therapy may be limited to very specific uses.

➤ If your plan does not offer alternative therapies and you choose to use them on your own, tell your primary care doctor (or specialist). Tell her what treatment you are receiving and who your provider is.

➤ If you don't check out your plan newsletter, you may be missing a whole host of classes, lectures, and support groups that help you maintain good health. They may also give you that important support you need during a serious illness.

➤ Your health plan save you money? It's possible. Check out the discounts and assistance your plan may offer for everything from health clubs to child care.

Part 5
Your Right to the Right Care

We've talked in this book about your health care "team," and your plan is likely to use this term, too. But every game has an umpire or ref to make sure everyone plays by the rules and the outcome is fair.

Managed care plans are no different. Most of the time (we hope), everybody on your health care team, from the doctor's receptionist to your surgeon to the plan's billing department, will be playing by the rules, and everybody will agree that the game's outcome is fair to everyone.

But sometimes different team members understand the rules differently. Other times they (intentionally or not) break the rules. And just to make things more complicated, sometimes the usual rules don't even apply.

In this section, we talk about how to find the right "ref" for your situation and how to make sure that your health care team plays by the rules.

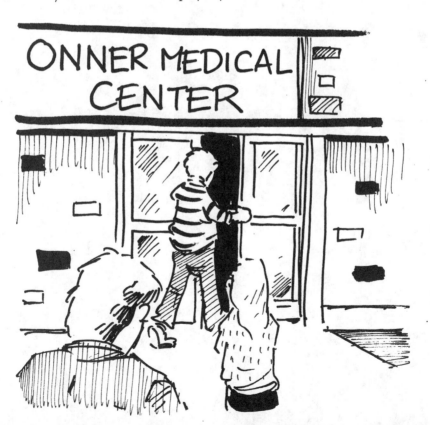

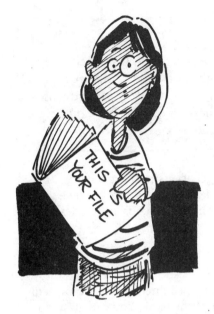

Chapter 22

Your Life on File

What do you see when you picture your medical record? Perhaps it's the school form that lists your vaccinations and how old you were when you had chicken pox. Maybe it's the three index cards your doctor writes your symptoms on in some indecipherable code every time he sees you. Or maybe it's a computer printout of dates and visits.

Now, picture a long and winding trail of footprints. You leave your footprint—your medical record—everywhere you receive medical care. But don't think there is an end to that trail, where the records of your illnesses, surgeries, and lab results reside neatly in one folder and are ready to be handed off to the next doctor. Your records reside wherever you get treatment. They are the caregiver's property. But the *information* in the records is yours.

House Call

There is no federal law regulating a patient's access to his or her own health records. State law varies widely. Some states don't allow you to see your own file, while others have laws that specifically cover the use and disclosure of health information. A little more than half of the states explicitly protect the rights of patients to review their records and to correct errors.

This chapter explains what is in your records, how you get access to those records, and who else can see all or part of the information in them. It also covers another type of information that is equally important to your care: your informed consent to a test or a procedure that is about to happen.

Who Wants to Know?

Because all your medical records aren't kept in one big filing cabinet, getting your medical information is not as easy as, say, getting money out of the bank. You can go to any ATM and get money from your account (provided there is money in the account), but you can't go across town and get your entire health care transferred immediately.

You have to ask that the information be sent to you or to someone else, like your primary care doctor. And your health care provider or managed care plan must have your permission to send your information somewhere else.

Big changes are afoot. On parallel tracks are the shift to managed care and the shift to keeping medical records electronically, with less and less kept on paper. In order to "manage" care, your health plan must bundle your information from everywhere you get service under the plan. Even networks bundle it more than in the past, though you are still required to ask that records be transferred from one doctor to the other.

With the explosive growth of both managed care and information technologies comes the reality that more people than you and your doctor have access to your medical records. Essentially, your doctor has two sets of customers: you and your managed care company.

There are a lot of reasons why many more people want and need your medical information. If your information is bundled with that of patients like you, with members of the same health plan, or members employed by the same employer, it provides powerful information on which to base treatments, guidelines, and negotiations between employers and health care plans.

What is your record used for? Your health care providers rely on it to plan your care. It also is used to verify billings and for health care research and planning.

We've talked in this book about the reliance on guidelines, how managed care companies use guidelines to follow your doctor's overall standard of care, and how medical services are delivered to their members. One of the ways plans develop and check the guidelines they use is by looking at patient data: your records along with all the other members. Your plan also uses this type of combined data as part of its quality assurance programs.

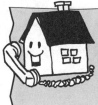

House Call

Pulling records for quality assurance is not a big source of patient privacy violations. Specific patient data is not part of quality assurance. It is designed to look at patterns of treatment or outcomes through combining the data on lots of members.

This is not much different from inventory management in a department store. If you have 300 pairs of one type of jeans sold over a week, you may get data on which sizes sold more than others, and, if credit cards are used, which ZIP codes really like that brand, and possibly how many are brought back with defects.

Health records are also used in federal enforcement actions. They are critical to the prosecution of health care fraud matters relating to medical necessity and improper billing under Medicare.

So now it is the payment system, the administration of health care, that drives the information system. The demand for information comes from outside the patient-doctor relationship; purchasers, payors, and consumers demand to know about the performance of health plans, doctors, hospitals, and others to make decisions. That information is based on your (and thousands of other patients') care.

Electronic records and data also make it faster and easier to get and give accurate information about the spread of disease, public health, and how well or poorly treatments and programs are meeting the needs of the public as well as plan members.

What Is in Your Medical Records?

Lots of things are in there. And if you can get a copy of your records, you may need some help deciphering them.

One way to get an idea of what is in your medical records is by using a list from the AHIMA. It suggests

Your Personal Rx

Get a copy of *Understanding Your Health Record*, available from the American Health Information Management Association (AHIMA). It is a professional organization representing experts who secure, analyze, and manage patient information. The publication lists documents common to most health records and common suffixes and prefixes to help interpret the medical terminology used. The association can be contacted at (312)787-2672 or **www.ahima.org**.

that when you request copies of your records, or are scheduled to see a new health care provider, request information such as:

➤ Problem list, including significant illnesses and surgeries

➤ Medication record, including prescriptions you've had and allergies to any of them

➤ Allergies list

➤ Immunization Report, including immunizations you have received and the dates

➤ Most recent history and physical

➤ Last year's progress notes, where your health care providers note your response to treatment and plans for continued treatment

➤ Lab, X ray, and scan reports

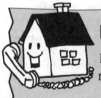

House Call

Many people are surprised to learn that your lab work typically will not include your blood type. If you give blood, the blood bank gives you a card with your type and has the information on file. If you don't know your blood type and want the information, ask the next time you have blood tests done.

➤ Consultation, or an opinion about your condition made by a doctor other than your primary care doctor. These would include second opinions.

➤ Operative reports, pathology reports, and discharge summaries. These are reports from hospital stays or surgeries. They are the who, what, when, where, and how (and result) of your hospital stay.

You can ask for a copy of your records and see if all this information is in them, or you can specify this list when you ask. You may get a copy of the full record, or you may get a summary. Keep it in a safe place.

House Call

Remember, your records are wherever you last left them. Unless you request that they be forwarded to your doctor, they don't get there.

You should have an idea of the accuracy of your records and what is being released when you authorize the disclosure of your records. Check that family history is recorded. If your records don't reflect an allergic reaction to penicillin, you can correct it. If your lab test or pathology report says more than your doctor told you about, you may want to talk to your doctor with your report in hand.

If you are having diagnostic tests, getting your records is essential to your understanding of what is going on. It allows you to view the reports, and it becomes more real to you.

Your record is also the legal document describing the care you received. If you challenge your health plan, or bring a complaint against the doctor, your record's accuracy (or the fact that it is inaccurate) is key.

If there are problems with information, they should be handled at the source, usually the physician's office. It is important for the patient to deal directly with the provider to ensure he is interpreting the information correctly. Decisions based on erroneous information may raise issues of liability. However, don't underestimate the difficulty of finding out where the "source" of the disputed information is; some elements of a record may originate at different sources. For information on fixing your medical records, start with your doctor; your plan's member services department may also be of help.

> **Your Personal Rx**
> Here's another reason to check your medical records. The Medical Information Bureau, an industry-supported clearing-house, keeps personal records used by insurance companies to make insurance determinations that affect health, life, and disability. There is a consent provision on most applications for insurance for release of information for these purposes. So check them out the same way you would your credit history.

Shhh: It's Private

The rapid move to electronic data is like the good twin and the evil twin. The good twin is the type of population-wide information that can lead to better care. The evil twin is the possibility of a breach of privacy, which may harm the person to whom the information pertains.

One of the areas people are concerned with is the chance that their employer will see their private medical records. It's true that more employers are asking for "good data" on their costs. The way to get it is to combine data of employees or members of the plan to show types of treatments, drugs, and therapies used and their costs.

The Medical Records Release

Most of us don't really know who has seen our medical records. We can guess, but we have little idea how many and who have access to our data when care is provided or claims are paid.

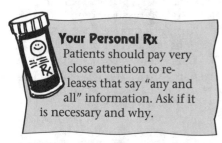

Healthspeak
Releases are current authorizations. You are allowing the medical information specified in the release to be given to whomever is specified. Sometimes information in a release is limited by state law.

When we sign a *release*, we rarely look at the document; it's just part of signing up for a health plan or getting treatment.

Hospitals are very controlled about who has access to medical records and are monitored by the states. Doctors' offices are not monitored the way hospitals are, however.

Before you sign a release for medical records, pay close attention to the following to make sure that only the necessary information (and no other) is released, and only to the right recipient:

➤ Name and institution to get the information

➤ Name of person or institution releasing it

➤ Patient's full name and date of birth

➤ A clear statement of the need for the information

➤ The extent of the information to be released and the date of treatment

➤ Date, event, such as a test or surgery, and when authorization expires

➤ The request should be retrospective not prospective; otherwise, it gives carte blanche for past, present, and future health information to be released.

Your Personal Rx
Patients should pay very close attention to releases that say "any and all" information. Ask if it is necessary and why.

Managed Care Plans and Your Files

In a managed care plan, information is released to whomever is working with the patient. It is part of the coordination of care. At that point in time, it has the patient's ID on it. The information is released on an as needed basis.

Managed care companies usually require full access to patient records, including those on mental health treatment. Companies require doctors to allow the plan to review their file as a condition to participate in the plan or to be reimbursed. This is an agreement signed between your mental health provider and the insurer. Some agreements go so far as to include notes taken during meetings with patients.

Information is also released to HEDIS (discussed in Chapter 6) and other data managers for the purpose of tracking patient care and outcomes. Such information has no patient identification.

Access and the Law

There is no comprehensive federal law that governs who has access to patient records or the reasons for accessing medical records. State laws are varied, weak, and inconsistent on matters pertaining to access to records, and haven't kept up with the information revolution. Whether and to what extent laws protect the confidentiality of health information also depends on who holds the information: doctor, hospital, health plan, or others.

HIPAA, the new federal act expanding health care coverage (see Chapter 7 for more on HIPAA), has criminal and civil penalties for those who knowingly disclose health information in violation of the act; this includes misuse of unique health identifiers (identifying information that can link you to your medical record) and obtaining individually identifiable health information.

House Call

Under the Health Insurance Portability and Accountability Act (HIPAA), there is no penalty for someone who discloses health information in violation of the act if the person did not know, and even with reasonable attentiveness would not have known, that he or she violated confidentiality provisions.

The following is a summary of how different states regulate the release of medical information.

➤ A majority of states impose on doctors and health care institutions the duty to maintain the confidentiality of medical records, but some do not. Slightly more than half extend this duty to other health care providers. But very few states impose this duty on insurers.

➤ A majority of states have penalties for unauthorized disclosure of health information. More provide civil than criminal penalties, and very few provide both.

➤ What about the duties of doctors and health care facilities? In some states, written authorization by the patient to permit disclosure by the provider does not allow further disclosure by the person who receives that information. In many states, information about mental health treatment may not be released without written, informed consent. States also require that facilities develop and implement policies designed to assure the security of patient information.

➤ Most states have laws forbidding psychiatrists and other mental health professionals from disclosing patient information except where authorized. But HMOs and other health plans require you to sign broad releases to get coverage. They can then give the information to interstate entities that are not subject to those laws.

Informed Consent

Informed consent gives hospitals and other medical facilities the right to treat the patient signing the form. Essentially, you are informed of the treatment to be performed, and your signature on the form is evidence that it was not performed against your will and without your consent. Don't sign an open consent, because that allows the hospital to do whatever it wants.

You may be asked to sign a consent form a number of times when you have surgery, tests, or other procedures, whether in a doctor's office or at the hospital. Read it, and make sure you understand it. If you don't, ask for explanations. Make sure you understand the risks. If you sign it, you are saying you understand what is in it and you understand the risks.

Don't be intimidated. If you have some lead time, ask to review the consent form in advance, and have someone review it with you. Bring someone along who can verify to you what you think is in the consent form, and make calls, if necessary, to get a clear understanding about what is to take place. Ask for written materials. You may want to tape record your discussions. People don't like it, but don't undervalue good preparation.

If you are faced with signing an informed consent form, ask these questions:

➤ What is the procedure or treatment?

➤ What are the risks and benefits? How often is the procedure successful: 90 percent of the time or 30 percent?

➤ Who will perform it?

➤ What are the side effects?

➤ What is the outcome if it is performed? What is the likely outcome if it is not performed?

➤ Are there any alternative treatments, and what are their risks and benefits?

See also Chapters 16, 17, and 18 for additional questions that may be appropriate to your particular circumstances.

Your Personal Rx
Many managed care plans are including classes on advance directives in their health education programs. Each state regulates the use of advance directives differently. The American Association of Retired Persons (AARP) has pamphlets available.

If you are participating in a clinical trial or other experimental treatment (see Chapter 18), you will be asked to sign an informed consent form. Ask the same questions as you would for any other informed consent form.

If you want to amend it and put in some extra terms or understandings, you can negotiate it. Remember, what you are consenting to should be explained to *your* satisfaction. After all, it's your body.

You should also be aware that you can give your family and any health care provider or facility instructions on what you want if the outcome is bad. An *advance directive* is instruction to health care facilities and family about what future medical care should be given, and what should not, in the event you become unable to speak for yourself.

The Least You Need to Know

➤ Records are the property of whomever gives you treatment, but the information is yours.

➤ Your health care records don't follow you along like a well-trained dog. You have to ask for them, and you have to ask for them to be sent to other places.

➤ You sign a release form when you join a managed care plan for those records to be released to whomever is giving you care in that plan.

➤ Your medical information, *without* your social security number, name, and other identification numbers, is bundled together with other members for many purposes.

➤ There is no federal law that governs who has access to patient records or the reasons for accessing those records. Confidentiality protections vary from state to state and may work differently from what you expect.

➤ All informed consent forms should be examined carefully before you sign them. Ask questions, and make sure that they are answered to *your* satisfaction.

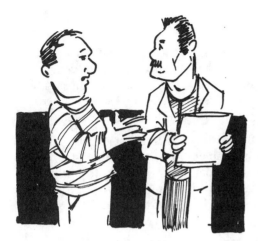

Chapter 23

When You Disagree: Working the System

> **In This Chapter**
>
> ➤ Reviewing your legal rights
>
> ➤ Picking the right person to talk to
>
> ➤ Filing a grievance
>
> ➤ Filing an appeal
>
> ➤ Dealing with arbitration
>
> ➤ Hiring a lawyer

We've talked throughout this book about your legal rights under your plan. They include, among other things, your right to a hearing when you feel you have been unfairly or wrongly denied treatment, and your right to use the courts to enforce your rights. This chapter is to help you protect these rights by explaining the procedures to follow when you disagree with your plan's decisions. If all the following suggestions fail, you'll unfortunately be reading Chapter 24 on how to wage a legal battle with your health care plan. But before you get to that point, read this chapter for information on how to deal with your problems in a less confrontational (and less costly) way.

Who Can Help—and When

You have friends, but, just as in your school playground, you have to learn how to pick them.

Talking to Member Services

This is not a formal procedure. It is the time, before any grievances are filed, for working things out. Most of the problems or questions you are likely to encounter with your managed care plan can probably be solved by a phone call to your doctor's or hospital's billing office or to the plan's member services or claims office. (See Chapter 17 for troubleshooting checklists).

Your Personal Rx
Member services will be keeping notes and records of calls and conversations, and you should, too. They may be very valuable if the situation escalates into something more confrontational.

If you are not satisfied with the results you get from member services, put your problem in writing and send it to the supervisor. The response may take two weeks to a month, so keep checking (but read Chapter 24 if you really have *no* time). Make sure you keep a copy of any letters you send to the plan.

If you are denied a claim, check out the following:

➤ Are the reasons for the denial ambiguous or vague? If so, write or call back (record your call but be sure to notify the other person you are doing so) and ask that it be explained to you more specifically.

➤ Ask what additional information or evidence you need to present to rebut the denial (see the discussion of billing, later in this chapter).

Remember, managed care plans are bureaucracies, no matter what they may want to call themselves, and they respond when you use their language. Refer to your member handbook and use the language you find there.

Your Doctor's Role

What if your doctor thinks your plan's decisions disagree with his medical judgment? He may be able to appeal to the utilization review (UR) body (see Chapter 2). When this happens, he needs to give you a careful explanation of why his recommended treatment is the best for the patient and the payor. Yes, that's right: What the doctor prescribes has to be good for your plan or insurance company as well, by saving money. This explanation should include:

➤ An explanation of the condition

➤ Reasons and expected benefits of the treatment, therapy, or test

➤ Alternatives to the proposed treatment, and why they are not right for the patient

➤ The risks of forgoing the recommended treatment, therapy, or test

Get any related documents, such as test results, used by the doctor in case you have to file a grievance or appeal a decision on your own.

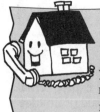

House Call

If your managed care plan continues to turn your request down and you decide to forgo care because of the expense involved, your doctor may ask you to sign an informed refusal that sets out why you have refused treatment.

Then the doctor should send a letter to the plan and the utilization review (UR) committee's chairperson with the same type of information listed above, the reason for his disagreement with the UR committee, and the problems that could result from failing to perform the recommended test or procedure. Get copies for yourself (all this should be in your medical record).

Can Your Employer or Insurance Agent Help?

If you have gone through the preceding steps with no luck, you may want to talk to your company's human resources office. Your employer may intercede with the plan if its decision violates the plan's terms (for instance, disallowing an emergency claim for a clear emergency) or if granting your request would not do so (for example, you want to choose a closer hospital for radiation treatment than the plan's contract hospital). Your employer may also step in even if the plan was right but communicated poorly with you.

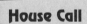

House Call

An employee fell ill during a business trip. The local doctor counseled immediate surgery, but the plan asked the employee to return home first. Worried, the employee had the surgery while away. When he filed for reimbursement, the plan initially refused. After discussions with the employer, the plan paid on the grounds that the employee's options and their consequences had not been adequately explained.

Human resources departments generally don't want to get in deep. They often try to steer you to the right person in the plan or to the right number to call. Some even assist in setting out what has to be in a letter to the plan. But many don't want to go further. When an employer buys the plan services, it doesn't like to second guess the way the plan works; that's part of the managed care plan's business acumen the employer buys. An employer's preference is to get the issues resolved, rather than get confrontational.

If you get your health coverage through an insurance agent, she can assist you in the grievance and appeals process. She can help write the grievance complaint or talk to the plan. She may also threaten to call the insurance commissioner and help the policyholder write to the commissioner, if necessary.

Two Little Words: "Experimental" and "Lawyer"

Most plans explicitly exclude from coverage any treatment considered experimental. Most of you reading this book are not scientists. You probably have little or no idea which treatments are experimental and which are widely accepted in the medical community for certain cases.

So avoid the word "experimental" in conversations, letters, or other communications with your employer or health care coverage plan. Be especially careful in signing informed consent forms for surgery; that fine print can hold a lot of important content (more on this in Chapter 22). If you want to convince your plan to cover something, you have to convince the plan that the treatment is *covered* under the terms of the plan, *not* that it falls into this prominent exclusion.

House Call

One patient signed an informed consent statement identifying her bone-marrow transplant for ovarian cancer as experimental. It was, as a matter of fact, performed as part of a clinical trial. She then sued the plan for reimbursement of her treatment costs. The court relied in part on the form she signed in ruling against her.

Making the case to your plan or insurance company about whether a given treatment is experimental or should be covered under the terms of the plan is best left to the professionals. Most doctors, clinics, and hospitals providing advanced treatments such as bone-marrow transplants retain on their staffs people who specialize in negotiating coverage with plans and insurance companies. They know how to present the scientific evidence supporting the recommendation of a particular patient for treatment.

As for the "L" word, *lawyer:* Never threaten anyone, especially in your company's personnel or human resources office. And don't mention a lawyer. We've often talked about the importance of allies in bureaucracies, including employers and health plans. Telling them you are getting a lawyer, or will do so if your needs are not met, raises the confrontation level, perhaps too early, and you may lose access to information you need to make your case, even though the information may be yours by right.

That doesn't mean you shouldn't contact a lawyer (more on lawyers later in this chapter). In fact, we think it's a good idea when there is a lot at stake. We just think that, tactically, it's better for the lawyer to decide when and how to contact the plan, because it will be part of the strategy to get you what you are entitled to.

Don't They Pay for This? Challenging a Bill

Unless you completely, intentionally flouted all the rules of the managed care plan, we suggest that you challenge a bill you think the plan is obligated to pay. Some plans may be overwhelmed by a surge in enrollment. Some may have other motives. But there are reports of many, many mistakes, with patients complaining they are being squeezed to pay doctors.

As we were writing this book, one of us received a bill from a hospital emergency room. She had taken her child there when he had a potentially fatal reaction to medication. Everyone who was supposed to be contacted—the primary care doctor and the plan—was contacted. And the emergency happened in a state that used the "prudent layperson" standard (see Chapter 14 for a definition). All in all, it was textbook perfect.

Three months after the incident, a bill arrived for the ER visit, and it was way beyond the copay. When the mom called member services, the representative told her the notation on the file stated that it was not an emergency. The author relayed all the events surrounding the trip, even explaining the state law (her anger was still under control). Everything fit the standard in the handbook. The member services rep then stated that she, too, was severely allergic to the same medication and knew it was an emergency. She then changed the billing code, and the next bill listed only the copay that was due.

You never know when, or why, you might make an ally.

It is always wise to check any medical bill you receive. And if you receive a bill from a doctor, therapist, hospital, or other facility that should be paid by your plan, check it out. Let your plan know if you see errors. Your plan may deny the claim, but it may also be for services neither you nor the plan incurred. Put your questions and findings in writing and keep copies. If you send a letter to a hospital or doctor, send a copy of it to your managed care plan (and keep one for yourself).

Filing a Grievance

What if you aren't able to resolve your conflict with the plan? You may be facing a task that is daunting but sometimes necessary: filing a *grievance*. Most grievance proceedings are slow and one sided. If you decide to go the grievance and appeal route, be prepared to know the levels of the game.

Members usually file grievances for either claims problems or service problems. Claims problems arise when you seek coverage not covered under the schedule of benefits, a treatment that is not considered medically necessary, or you are denied or reduced coverage for services already incurred. This may occur even if you followed the rules and got the authorization.

Service problems arise for issues that involve the quality of care, such as your inability to get timely appointments or difficulty getting referrals. Administrative problems, such as incorrect ID cards or lack of plan updates, may also be included.

A grievance is usually handled in-house. That means everyone who handles the grievance—member services, the medical director, counsel—is employed by the plan.

What Should You Do?

You can find information on filing a grievance in your member handbook. However, most we've seen did not have the nuts-and-bolts of filing a grievance and what it entails.

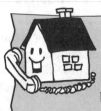

Healthspeak

A *grievance* is a complaint that something happening in your health plan is unjust, does not meet the terms of the plan, or causes injury. A grievance is a formal procedure. State and federal regulations require that HMOs have clearly defined grievance procedures. We've found them less than clear.

Call member services and ask them how to submit a written grievance. Ask if they have any written information on filing a grievance and have them send it to you. You may want to call twice to make sure you get the same information each time. We've had conflicting information on grievances when we've called plans. If the information is not the same each time, ask for the supervisor. These are the types of calls you may want to record (don't forget to notify the other party!), or at least take detailed notes on who answered the call, date, and what was said. When you become more confrontational, more "rules" seem to appear.

Make sure to get answers to the following questions before you proceed with a grievance:

➤ How do I file a grievance and to whom is it addressed?

➤ What information should be contained in the letter?

➤ How long do I have to file a grievance from the time of the denial or incident?

➤ How long does the health plan have to respond to me? It may be 30 days for federal employees and 60 days for others. It depends on what is in the contract between the employer (or individual) and the plan.

➤ Who do I call to find out the status of my grievance?

➤ If I am not satisfied, whom do I contact in the organization about an appeal?

House Call

In a point-of-service plan, a claim for unauthorized services is considered to be out-of-network, so there is no claim problem. It is viewed basically as a voluntary self-referral. You just have to pay more than you would if the services were authorized.

Each plan has different requirements for what you need to put in a grievance filing, but here are the main points yours should contain:

➤ Name and membership number on your card

➤ Who is involved (name of doctor, hospital, or other provider of health care)

➤ Narration of events: who, what, when, where, how, what they said, and dates

➤ Responses by parties and dates

➤ If you asked for information and were denied, if you were promised follow-up either by phone or mail and you did not receive it, and dates

Watch time limits on when you can file a grievance. If the problem arose in January, for instance, and you wait until October to file, you may have lost your right to file a grievance. If you aren't getting any satisfaction through informal channels, or your ability to prevail is iffy, file a grievance before your time limit is up. Your informal complaints to member services may not stay your time.

Your Personal Rx
Always ask if the plan has an expedited complaint and appeals process. This process is usually reserved for patients with life-threatening conditions.

Be prepared to wait. Some plans promise to take from 30 to 60 days to make a decision, but it is often much longer. During that time, the plan is expected to investigate the claim, conducting interviews and collecting any other pertinent information.

At the end of this period, you will (or should) receive a response with findings and what is finally resolved. If you are not satisfied, you must respond back to the plan within a certain time period.

Your Personal Rx
If you've filed a grievance in one plan, don't assume the process is the same in another plan. Each plan has its own way of doing things.

Special Rules for Medicare

If you use Medicare, the federal government requires that your managed care plan have special rules for grievances. They provide for a much faster review than is usually the case for members.

The HMO must accept an oral request for a review, give prompt notice as to whether the review will be expedited (on the fast track), and notify you of the decision within 72 hours after the request. It must accept a doctor's request for an expedited review regardless of whether the doctor is affiliated with the HMO.

If the request is denied, you have the right to have the decision reconsidered, including an expedited reconsideration under the same procedures and same time frame as the first review.

If you are denied care after the appeal, you can take your case directly to Medicare. It will be reviewed by a panel of medical experts. Urgent cases will be reviewed within three days. If you lose here, you can take it to an administrative judge (a judge in the Department of Health and Human Services).

Appeals

All insurers have financial incentives to discourage appeals of their administrative decisions. The appeals process costs money and, if the decision goes your way, it will cost them more money. That's why appealing correctly and having some professional help can be worthwhile.

Your Personal Rx

Plans set the time period for requesting both appeals and reviews. If you miss that filing time, you may lose your opportunity. But the plan also has a certain amount of time in which to respond to your request, so watch the calendar and hold them to that limit.

You have the right to appeal. But you have to request it; it does not happen automatically. The appeal may be handled by a senior person in the health care plan or by someone outside the plan.

Sometimes, third-party medical experts review certain denials of medical procedures, though these experts are picked by the plans. Stories abound on medical experts who simply write the same denial with the same reasoning again and again—regardless of the facts in the case.

Make sure you find out how your plan handles appeals. Usually, the first appeal is "on the record," which means that it is based on the files of the case, rather than testimony or formal hearings. But some plans allow formal hearings, so it's important to find out exactly what happens under your plan.

If you do have a formal hearing, this is where you make your case. Fair warning: You are probably making your case to people employed by the plan, though not necessarily the people who have been involved in your dispute.

Remember that second opinion? If your second opinion differs from that of the experts hired by your plan, get that second opinion on the record in your hearing, with any other supporting documents, such as lab tests.

Don't expect to receive a finding that day. You will be told that you will receive the results within a certain amount of time, for example, ten working days. Be sure to keep checking to make sure the plan holds to this promise.

Generally, you may be prohibited by your (or your employer's) contract with the health plan from filing a lawsuit over benefits denial until you have gone through the plan's grievance procedures (but see Chapter 24 for some important exceptions to this requirement), including appeals.

If you are a federal employee, you have the right to appeal to the Office of Personnel Management (OPM). OPM specifically reserves the right in its contracts with managed care plans to rule on grievances by members who are federal employees.

If you are on Medicare or Medicaid, you also have special appeal rights. Medicare members have the right to appeal to the Health Care Financing Administration (HCFA), and Medicaid members can appeal to state welfare departments.

> **House Call**
>
> A few states have external appeals processes for patients denied medical procedures by their HMO. Some are limited to very specific areas, like experimental treatment. You still have to go through the managed care appeals process before moving to the state for action. Review there may be by a peer review organization, made up of doctors, or an impartial, national expert.

Arbitration

Some plans require you to submit disputes to *arbitration*. If you belong to a plan through your employer, it's in the contract between your employer and the managed care plan. If you get it individually, it's in the contract between you and the plan.

In arbitration, a dispute is settled by a person or persons chosen to hear both sides and come to a decision.

And if you try to strike it from a contract for individual coverage, you may get turned away from the health plan.

Make sure you watch for notifications of changes in your plan that require arbitration for certain issues. You may miss them in the materials you get from the plan, and it is important to know.

> **Healthspeak**
>
> *Arbitration* is a dispute resolution process involving a hearing outside a court. The arbitrators, who are supposed to be neutral, hear a complaint and resolve the dispute. That resolution is final and binding on all parties.

Arbitration is different from court proceedings. The insurance company or health care plan will be represented by a lawyer, usually one who depends on the company for a living. You, on the other hand, will be represented by a doctor and will have an attorney present only if you decide to do so. There will also generally be an outside doctor on the panel. The health plan may use an independent arbitration service or individual lawyers trained in arbitration. Some managed care plans run their own system.

In court, on the other hand, the judge is bound by clear rules and precedents, and doesn't depend on either of the parties for a livelihood. And, unlike arbitration, the results of a court case are subject to appeal.

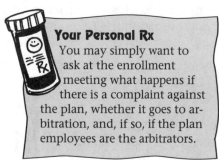

Your Personal Rx
You may simply want to ask at the enrollment meeting what happens if there is a complaint against the plan, whether it goes to arbitration, and, if so, if the plan employees are the arbitrators.

If you lose at arbitration, you usually can't make your case in court. Over the last ten years, courts have broadened the scope of arbitration and take a dim view of reviewing an arbitrator's decisions. The results of an arbitration proceeding are binding on both parties and are reviewable by a court only for gross—that means serious—errors. The presumption, should you go to court, is that the results of the arbitration will be upheld unless something really bad happened in the process. For instance, if the plan treats arbitration as a sham or makes a practice of long delays even though the contract says "speedy" or "expeditious," it may be sued for fraud.

Fortunately, even if your plan provides for binding arbitration, you may be able to go to court instead. Your day in court is the subject of Chapter 24.

Do I Need a Lawyer?

You can file a grievance yourself, especially if you're contesting a relatively small claim. But if the treatment you are seeking is important to your life and health or that of a loved one, or the sum of money involved is large, you should probably get a lawyer involved early. The reason is simple: You could lose. If the grievance is denied, and the issue is important enough to you, you'll need to appeal (see above), and eventually you may end up in court. You want to have the early, formal procedures done right for you in case you have to go to court later, when those earlier filings become critical.

Your grievance or appeal letter has to contain all the information you would use in court if you had to. As one experienced attorney told us, the letter has to have all the reasons why you're right and they're wrong. But unless you are an attorney yourself—and perhaps not even then—you are unlikely to be able to preview an entire court case in the course of one letter. It's best to hire an attorney, but only if the amount at stake warrants the legal fees.

How to Talk to a Lawyer: It's Easier Than You Think!

It's extremely important to find out if the attorney has experience with health care coverage and benefit denials. The lawyer who handled your will, divorce, or real estate closing may be a competent professional and even a close friend. However, the more competent your attorney is, the better that person will understand that appealing a health care treatment decision can be a matter of life and death for you. Therefore, it should be handled by a specialist. If you get the treatment you need and live to talk about it, you can always take your lawyer out to lunch and apologize.

Here's a script you can follow:

➤ Introduce yourself. Briefly explain the problem: your diagnosis or medical condition, the treatment (or payment for treatment you have received) you want, the steps you have gone through already, the results to date.

➤ Ask the attorney, "Do you handle cases such as mine?"

➤ If the answer is "Yes," ask, "How many have you handled? How many have you won?" (This is your life at stake, here. It's not the time to worry about some stranger's ego.)

➤ If the conversation has gone well to this point and you are interested in retaining the attorney, ask, "Will there be a charge for the initial review of my case?" If you are going to an expert in the field, you will usually not be charged for this initial review. But if there is a charge, find out if it is hourly or for the whole review (which could take several hours).

➤ You may also want to ask what the attorney expects your case to cost. An appeal to the plan will cost you , but you may be awarded attorneys' fees at the plan's expense if you win in court (see Chapter 24). Ask about his experience with attorneys fees.

Attorneys who represent people in health care disputes know they are dealing with sick and frightened people. They should understand if you are stressed out. But stay calm enough to assess an attorney's competence and help the attorney win your case. If you have gotten satisfactory answers to the questions we list above, you should be well on the way to a cooperative and successful relationship.

What Your Lawyer May Need

Whether it's to file a grievance or an appeal or to take your plan to court, the attorney will need the following documents:

➤ Summary of your health status (if you have been recommended for a bone-marrow transplant or similar treatment, your medical team has done such a summary)

➤ A copy of your health care plan documents

➤ Copies of your correspondence with the plan or health care providers

The attorney will write a detailed letter explaining your case and include any materials that support your claim. He will focus on explaining why the treatment should be covered under the terms of the plan, so be sure to bring him all the information you can about how the plan is actually run.

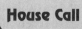

House Call

The initial consultation with the attorney is usually free, but you should ask. Depending on the business climate in your area, attorneys could charge several hundred dollars an hour for evaluating your case. Find out if there are other fees, such as court costs or travel costs for the attorney or experts, that you will have to pay up front.

The Least You Need to Know

➤ Stay calm. You are less likely to miss an important step.

➤ Your HR department can point you in the right direction, but it won't want to get in deep when you and your plan have a dispute.

➤ If you don't think you owe the bill in your hand, don't pay it until you check it out with the plan, hospital, or doctor.

➤ Find out everything you can about your grievance and appeals proceedings and keep excellent records of any calls, letters, and documents.

➤ Arbitration is not like court; there are fewer rules and protections. But even if your plan provides for arbitration, you may be able to make your case in court instead.

➤ You do not need an attorney to appeal a treatment decision by your plan, but it's a good idea to have one if a lot is at stake. An attorney's advice can help you win the appeal—and safeguard your rights in court if you lose the appeal.

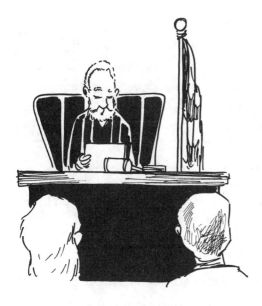

Court as a Last Resort

Your lawyer may one day become one of your health care professionals. Your lawyer may not even know how to administer an aspirin, but there could come a time when he or she could be the most important person on your health care team.

We never gave you instructions for performing your own (or a loved one's) brain surgery. We just gave you information on how, if you needed brain surgery, to get the right care in a managed care system. Here, we don't tell you how to be your own lawyer when you're not getting the right care and court is your last resort. We just tell you what you should be aware of if you need to get a lawyer and go to court.

This chapter is for people who need treatment their plan is not willing to provide and who have gone through all the steps we listed in Chapters 17 and 23. In this chapter, we talk about what happens if you have to go to court to get the care you need. But remember—you go through the steps listed in Chapters 17 and 23 first.

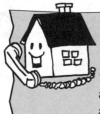

House Call

We discussed hiring an attorney in Chapter 23; the process is the same whether you are hiring an attorney to file a plan appeal, to go through arbitration, or to head for court. Check that chapter, too, for pitfalls to avoid in any dispute with your plan.

A caveat: While you may be able to get around your plan's appeal or arbitration rules, *never* skip asking the plan for preauthorization for treatment, even if you think the preauthorization will be denied. Skipping this step could be used against you if you have to go to court.

Following the Rules—or Not

We've said many times in this book that the managed care mantra is "Rules rule."

And we've also been telling you that "There are rules, and then there are rules."

You must generally follow the plan's administrative procedures to appeal a treatment or reimbursement decision. These rules are specified in the plan. The rules are designed to keep you out of court as long as possible, possibly forever. However, the law does not require that you *always* exhaust *all* administrative procedures before going to court.

There are two prominent exceptions to this requirement that your plan will not tell you about:

➤ You do not have to follow all the plan's administrative procedures—including arbitration—if you have reason to believe it is futile to do so. Your belief must be solidly based in fact and data, not just intuition. You could think following the arbitration rules, for example, is futile because you have been told by someone in a position of authority in your company or your health insurance plan, "The company (or the plan) will never approve this operation." Or the plan may have denied a number of other such requests as yours in the past.

➤ You do not have to follow the rules in an emergency. Unlike a visit to the emergency room, you don't have to be in immediate danger of death when certain administrative rules are concerned. You only have to have less time available to make a decision than the plan requires to make a decision on your appeal. Some plans now give themselves 30 days but many give themselves 90 days or more to respond to an appeal of a treatment decision. But in cancer treatment, for example, you may have to undertake treatment within six weeks of your surgery. That treatment, in turn, may have to be scheduled by your hospital or doctor, further reducing the time you have available to make your decisions. You also may not have much time to spare in a problem pregnancy.

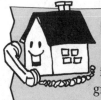

House Call

If your plan offers an expedited hearing on your appeal, you may find it difficult to bypass your plan's arbitration requirement on emergency grounds. Talk to an experienced lawyer and give her all the facts.

When Time Is Not on Your Side

You're sick, and you're scared. Your attorney thinks you have a good shot in court, but you'd rather spend your time getting care, even if it's not the care you feel you need. You're worried that going to court will leave you both poorer and less able to benefit from treatment than if you took your chances with arbitration.

Is court or arbitration better for you?

Everything depends on your individual circumstances, including your health, but don't assume that going to court will waste valuable time that you could otherwise spend getting treatment. One experienced attorney told us that with a legitimate emergency, an attorney can file suit "right away." In one case, he filed suit on a Thursday and was in court on the following Monday.

And don't discount the possibility that once it becomes clear you're willing to go to court, the plan will become willing to negotiate. In fact, try to hire a lawyer who is willing to negotiate creatively.

House Call

In one dispute over a bone-marrow transplant, an insurance company made a donation to a foundation that then paid for the transplant. This solution allowed the insurer to continue to say that it had never paid for a transplant. This solution didn't help the next patient, but it sure helped the person whose life was on the line.

When to Sue

Only your attorney—after consulting with your doctor—knows for sure. If you have time, you can negotiate, or you can pursue the plan's administrative procedures. If you don't have time, such as when an emergency evolves into a head to head dispute with the hospital or plan and you, you may want to telephone your attorney right away.

> **House Call**
>
> Sometimes court may be your *first* step, because there is literally *no* time to waste. Under federal law, for example, a hospital may not discharge or transfer a patient unless the patient is "stable." *Stability*, unfortunately, has been interpreted in a number of ways. One Colorado hospital discharged a woman suffering from an infection by "flesh-eating" bacteria. The patient, of course, died.

> **Healthspeak**
>
> An *injunction* is a court order requiring that someone or something perform a particular act, or refrain from performing a particular act. There are different types of injunctions, depending on what you are asking for and what must finally be resolved.

Even if your plan has agreed to finance your treatment, your struggle may not be over. Plans have canceled preapproved procedures as late as the eve of the surgery. If your coverage is under an employer-sponsored plan, you have none of the legal protections you would if you had a contract to buy a house or a refrigerator. All you can do is stay in touch with your attorney.

If you are asking the plan to specifically *do*, or not do, something, your attorney may go into court and ask for an *injunction*.

Where to Sue

The U.S. court system has different levels. In a health care coverage dispute, you may sue in either federal or state court. Federal and state courts often take different types of cases and decide them in different ways.

Where you end up will generally depend on where you are in the treatment process. If you are suing to get the plan to adhere to the terms of its agreement with your employer, state and federal courts typically have concurrent jurisdiction; that means your lawyer could sue in either place. Generally, most of this type of litigation takes place in federal court.

House Call

If your health care coverage is as a federal, state, or local government employee or the dependent of one, you may have more extensive rights in a dispute with your plan than those available to private-sector employees. But in such a dispute, you should proceed in much the same way: Read and understand your plan documents, and consult an attorney who has experience in your type of plan.

What to Sue For

Your health plan has hurt (or refused to help) you, or so you feel. You're mad, and someone has to pay. How much? In what form? There are rules on this, and the rules are much different from what happens if you slip on your neighbor's icy sidewalk or eat a bad burrito at the local beanery. Let's look at the possible scenarios.

What if you've had bad, injurious medical treatment? Or bad decisions have left you injured because you did not get the right treatment? Medical malpractice is a state issue. Right now, in most states, your health plan can't be held liable for malpractice. You can get only the cost of treatment (plus legal fees) if the court agrees with you that the plan should have paid. Malpractice claims are generally filed against health care providers.

HMOs usually argue that malpractice does not apply to them, only to the physician. The physician usually works for them under some type of contract and so may be an independent contractor. The HMO is protected by ERISA from malpractice claims because it is involved in the administration of health care, not actually "providing" health care. It sounds as though all the HMO does is move paper from one side of the desk to the other, but it does much more. That's the conundrum. Even when it exercises judgment on whether care is medically necessary, its decisions are considered benefit decisions made in the course of managing employee benefit plans.

Healthspeak
The Employee Retirement Income Security Act (ERISA), the federal law that regulates employee benefit plans, generally *preempts* state laws, insofar as they apply to private-sector employee benefit plans. For instance, state insurance laws can't be enforced against an employee benefit plan, even if the state law sets a higher standard of benefits than available in the plan. This is one of the most difficult areas to understand. It is essential that your attorney understand it.

Caution
Beware of any attorney who promises you the moon in a health care coverage lawsuit because you are suing a company with "deep pockets." If your coverage is through an employer-sponsored plan, those pockets are mostly sewn shut if you have to sue in federal court under ERISA.

House Call

Two federal circuit courts have held that HMOs can be held liable for malpractice. These circuits cover Delaware, New Jersey, Pennsylvania, Colorado, Kansas, New Mexico, Oklahoma, Utah, and Wyoming. In addition, Texas has become the first state in the nation to pass a law allowing managed care organizations to be held legally liable for negligent medical decisions.

When You Might Get Treatment and Legal Expenses

In the best of possible worlds, if you have to go to court, you will be suing for treatment before the denial of treatment has hurt your health. If the court agrees that, by the terms of the plan, the plan was supposed to cover your treatment, you will get the cost of treatment.

You may get your costs of fighting the case, at the judge's discretion. Be sure to ask your attorney if she has received payment of legal expenses in previous cases of your type.

But even if your health has already been harmed by the denial of treatment—say, your cancer was diagnosed too late for effective treatment—you might be able to get only the cost of the treatment the plan should have paid for. Suppose the plan denied you a $100 test for cancer. You paid for the test yourself, but, by then, the cancer was too advanced for treatment. In court, you should be able to recover the cost of the test. That's it. You will not get money damages for pain and suffering.

When You Might Get Damages

If your doctor diagnoses your case incorrectly, makes a mistake in treating you, fails to tell you about a treatment that could help you, or fails to protest your plan's denial of treatment he or she has recommended, you can still sue your doctor for malpractice, individually, in state court. But the plan is responsible only if you live in one of the states where the courts or state laws have held them so.

You may get money to cover the damage the doctor has done to you as well as punitive damages, intended to deter the doctor from doing it again. You might also get reimbursed for your legal expenses in this case as well.

When You Might Get Nothing

Yes, nothing. You may have been denied treatment by your plan, resulting in lasting harm to you. There may be no dispute that the plan's decision caused this harm. Yet you might get nothing in court.

One HMO patient had a high-risk pregnancy. Her doctor wanted to hospitalize her close to her due date. The plan refused but placed a nurse in the patient's home for 10 hours a day. The problem was, the patient lost the baby when the nurse was off duty.

The patient sued the plan for damages. Guess what? She didn't get anything! Because she had not been hospitalized—the plan had refused—there were no hospital costs to pay. Because nothing had been done for the patient, there was nothing for her to recover in court. And because she was suing in *federal* court—she had to—she could not allege medical malpractice by the plan.

> **House Call**
>
> If your plan denies you care your doctor feels is medically necessary, you may be able to get the care on credit. Then, and only then, would you be able to recover anything from the plan. However, if the court decides that the plan acted correctly, either you or the institution that took care of you would be stuck with a large unpaid health care bill.

Whom to Sue

Depending on your circumstances, you might be able to sue your employer, your plan, your doctor, or your insurance company. Whom you should sue will generally depend on the nature of your problem and the kind of plan you have.

Your employer has legal obligations to you, such as telling you about the plan and changes. But anyone in a decision-making position with respect to the plan may be responsible for discharging certain obligations, such as notifying you of your right to continue coverage after you are no longer covered under a group plan (see Chapter 7 for more on this).

While these rules are not necessarily rocket science, how they are applied may depend on the specific contracts, responsibilities, and agreements surrounding your plan. This is just another reason for consulting an attorney who specializes in health care coverage issues, and for asking careful questions about what he or she thinks went wrong in your case (and thus who is responsible for making it right).

> **Your Personal Rx**
> Believe it or not, sometimes attorneys sue the wrong entity (in one case, the insurance company when the employer was at fault). Good attorneys know what is going on all over the country. Ask your attorney about cases similar to yours and how they turned out. If you don't get an answer or don't understand it, get a second opinion or change attorneys.

What It's Worth to You

Health care costs are astronomical. Legal fees haven't quite gotten there yet, but they're pretty high as well.

Attorneys' hourly rates vary widely among communities. More experienced attorneys might well charge more than those who are less experienced. If you have a serious health-related legal problem, this might not be the time to pinch pennies.

In the Washington, D.C., area, where we live, retaining an attorney experienced in insurance matters for a preliminary court hearing may cost you $15,000; a trial $30,000 to $50,000. This is serious money, but remember: If you win, you may get your legal costs as well. Hiring an attorney for an appeal or arbitration should cost less than for a court hearing but, as we've said before, feel free to ask.

The Least You Need to Know

➤ As a managed care plan member, you are obligated to follow the plan's administrative rules if you disagree with its decision. But there are two exceptions to this requirement that no one's going to tell you about. You can bypass some of the rules if you have good reason to think it's futile to follow them or if you have a medical emergency.

➤ Even in an emergency, always ask the plan for preauthorization of the care you want. Not doing so could cost you later.

➤ Don't expect to make big bucks by suing your health care plan. In most cases, the best you can hope for is the cost of treatment plus legal fees. In some cases, you might not even get that.

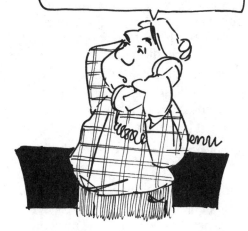

Chapter 25

UH-HUH. WHERE IN SOUTH AMERICA DID YOU STUDY MEDICINE?

Who's Minding the Store: Regulation and Accreditation

In This Chapter

➤ Your plan answers to a higher authority—maybe

➤ When to call the feds

➤ When to call the state

➤ When you're on your own

Your managed care plan has taken on the responsibility of watching you, your doctor, your hospital, and your employer to see that its standards for cost-effective care are met.

But who's watching your plan?

Your plan has the power to affect your health, your doctor's livelihood, and your hospital's solvency. Who makes sure it follows its own rules, let alone the rules of the federal and state governments? Where can you go if you think your plan is slipping up?

It depends. Some plans may have lots of people watching over *their* shoulders as they watch you. Others slip through the cracks, and you, the consumer, may not always be able to tell.

In this chapter, we tell you how to get help from the people your plan has to answer to.

The Regulatory Lineup

Federal and state governments generally share responsibility for regulating health plans. But there's sharing, and there's sharing.

If you're a parent, you share responsibility for your children's care and discipline with your spouse (at least that's the way it works in theory). You uphold each other's rules. Mom says no ice cream before dinner? Dad says the same thing. And if one of you is away from home or out of town, the other takes over the missing parent's responsibilities. Dad sees to his daughter's ponytail; Mom pitches a few balls for front-yard softball practice.

But suppose the kids could get ice cream before dinner as long as they asked Mom and not Dad. Or suppose only Mom could fix her daughter's hair, or only Dad could toss the ball around with Junior. Seems like it could lead to a lot of loose hair and loose balls.

This setup is much like the way the federal and state governments "share" the regulation of health plans:

> ➤ The federal government regulates federal and private-sector employee benefit plans. Most people under age 65, and a lot of those 65 and older, get their coverage through such plans. The federal government does not, however, regulate insurance companies, even though many employee benefit plans are offered through insurance companies.

> ➤ The states regulate insurance companies and the plans and policies they offer. They also license doctors, hospitals, and other health care providers. The states do not regulate employee benefit plans, other than those for their own employees, even though providing such benefits is many insurance companies' major reason for being.

Many health care plans that cover private-sector employees and their families have to live in both worlds. So, like the kids in our hypothetical family, they have to figure out both their parents' rules.

On the one hand, both insured and self-insured plans have to follow the federal tax code's rules about how employee benefit plans are run. Otherwise, they risk losing both the employer's and the employee's ability to avoid paying taxes on premiums paid for health care coverage.

It's a different story when it comes to complying with insurance laws. The U.S. Supreme Court has held that only insured plans—those funded through insurance policies—are subject to state insurance laws. These laws mandate anything from solvency requirements and premium rates to the types of benefits the plans they sell must offer. These benefits can include anything from chiropractic care to well-baby care to infertility treatments to bone-marrow transplants.

Self-insured plans—those in which the employer pays for claims out of its own funds rather than buying an insurance policy—are not subject to state laws, though many might offer the same benefits required under state law. They're subject only to ERISA, which is not an insurance law, but one aimed at safeguarding employee benefit rights.

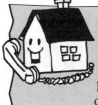

House Call

For some complaints, like safety violations, dangerous employees, or unprofessional conduct at work, it doesn't matter what type of health plan you have. You can, and should, complain to the appropriate board or health and safety department.

But wait—there's more. The Supreme Court has also ruled that health insurers are exempt from state laws allowing juries to assess punitive damages if an insurer has improperly denied a claim. These claims must therefore be argued in federal court. After you get to federal court, all you, the plaintiff, can get is the cost of the treatment (sometimes; see Chapter 24 for an explanation) and, at the court's discretion, legal fees (that's only if the court agrees with you).

House Call

Our hypothetical ACHES Plan, which is insured, has to offer state-mandated benefits, but PANES Plan, a self-insured plan in the same state, does not. But if either plan improperly denies a benefit to a member, it can be forced to pay only for the benefit. It can't be punished for its decision, however negligent—and harmful—its benefit denial may have been (see Chapter 24 for more on this).

How do you know whether your plan answers to the feds, your state, or both?

Even experts get confused. You and your neighbor may be getting care from the same health plan, but his policy is through an insured plan, and yours is through your employer's self-insured plan.

How can you find which one you have? If your coverage is through an employer, the first place you should look to find out whether your plan is insured is your Summary Plan Description (or SPD, described in Chapter 3). You got one when you signed up in your employer's health plan. If you can't find the answer in the SPD, call your employer's human resources office and ask which type of plan you have. Remember to be clear about the plan you're enrolled in; some employers offer both insured and self-insured plans, often with similar names.

Don't call the insurance company where you send your claims. The people in the customer service department are unlikely to know, as any insurance company may run lots of different types of benefit plans under lots of different arrangements.

> ### House Call
>
> If you are buying your health care coverage on your own and do not have coverage through an employer plan—COBRA coverage (explained in Chapter 7) doesn't count—you are in an insured plan. Your plan has to obey all applicable state insurance laws, and you can sue it in state court.

The Feds

Two federal agencies share most of the federal regulation of employee benefit plans: the U.S. Department of Labor and the Internal Revenue Service (IRS). If you believe your federal benefit rights have been violated, you can call either agency at the number listed in the federal government section of your telephone directory.

In general, the Labor Department is concerned with enforcing participants' benefit rights. The IRS is concerned with making sure employers adhere to the tax code rules that allow them to sponsor—and deduct the costs of—employee benefit plans. You may not easily be able to decide which heading your problem falls under, however. Let the pros make the decision; call both.

The federal Equal Employment Opportunity Commission (EEOC) is responsible for enforcing the Americans with Disabilities Act (ADA), including the act's employee benefit provisions. If you feel you have been discriminated against in access to health care coverage based either on a disability or on someone's perception that you have a disability, the EEOC may be able to help. Again, check the federal government listings in your local telephone directory.

When the State Steps In

State insurance commissioners like to know what is happening in their jurisdiction. The following are some of the issues that state insurance regulators must consider.

Can It Bear the Risk?

One of the big concerns of state insurance regulators is to make sure that you get what you pay for. You pay your premiums, and your plan is obligated to pay for what it promises in the contracts. But health care coverage is a risky business. If an insurer charges each insured person $3,000 for a year's coverage, it hopes (and plans) that each person costs it somewhat less. The difference between the two is the firm's profit.

But what if the average person incurs $3,300 in medical claims? Yes, someone may lose his or her job for not making the right calculations. But you shouldn't lose health care coverage you paid for. That's the responsibility of insurance regulators. One of their main jobs is to make sure that the company can pay for the health care its members have paid for even if the company has miscalculated its expenses. Otherwise, there would be nothing to protect you from the unscrupulous (or incompetent) company that undercuts the competition at, say, $2,000 per person, then folds when it can't pay the claims that come in.

The states regulate insurance companies, as well as any entity that is not actually licensed as one but bears risk. The latter group includes HMOs. These entities have to be licensed by the state just to do business, so even if they do not have to observe many state insurance laws, they have to behave to get and keep their licenses.

Other HMO Issues Regulated by States

There are other issues that states regulate. Most states set a limit on an HMO's reach to a designated service area, usually by ZIP code or county. Such limits prevent HMOs from marketing their services to people in areas they are not equipped to serve. Most also require HMOs to hold open enrollment periods. And some states require quality assurance standards. This may include a requirement to report grievances filed and processed by the HMO on a regular basis.

More states are passing laws that give stronger consumer protections for members of HMOs. A number of states, including Ohio, Florida, Texas, Minnesota, and New York, have passed comprehensive consumer rights laws affecting managed care. Watch your newspaper and local news reports for reports of new consumer legislation that take on health care.

Utilization review (UR) organizations, whether independent of HMOs or within the plan, may fall under state regulation. A little more than half the states have laws that require certain rules be followed and that individuals or corporations that do UR be licensed. However, ERISA protects UR organizations from state regulation if they contract exclusively with self-funded plans.

> **Your Personal Rx**
> States are providing more consumer assistance on insurance issues. For instance, the Washington State Office of the Insurance Commissioner staffs a consumer hot line 12 hours a day. You can use the hot line to obtain complaint forms or even launch an official investigation of your complaint. You can also get brochures and fact sheets.

PPOs

Nobody regulates PPOs, however. That's right—nobody. Most states do not regulate quality assurance activities for PPOs, and, if they do, the regulations are less stringent than those applied to HMOs. But if you are covered under a PPO and the plan is insured, the state regulates the insurance company that sponsors your plan or contracts with the PPO to serve its policy holders. In a PPO, therefore, if you have a problem, you go to the state insurance regulators for help.

Neither Fish nor Fowl: Plans at the Regulatory Frontier

Remember what we told you in Chapter 18 about the frontiers of medical research? There are fewer rules, and things can get pretty wild.

The same is true of plans at the frontiers of managed care. What you have to remember about managed care is that it's a relatively new industry. New forms of doing business are emerging all the time. When they do, government regulation may not always be there to greet them.

> **House Call**
>
> There are real limits to state investigatory agencies. There are limits on the power they wield and on the resources they have, and they simply don't adapt as quickly as the organizations they are required to watch over.

States are just finding their way on how to treat new entities such as provider networks—groups of doctors, hospitals, and other health care providers—that, by their financing arrangements, are bearing risk. Integrated service networks, physician-hospital organizations, and provider cooperatives are examples of such networks. As in the insurance company example above, they are taking premiums and hoping that those premiums cover the cost of their customers' care.

Many such networks contract directly with employers or groups of employers, thereby bypassing the health plan "middle man." Cutting out another player can bring financial benefits to both the employer and the network. But the catch for you, the plan member, can be that they are also cutting out some of the regulatory players as well. While an HMO that offers its services to lots of different customers has to be licensed by the state to do business, a provider network that functions like an HMO but offers its services directly to only certain employers may not have to.

One school of thought is that such provider networks become engaged in the business of insurance when they assume risk, and thus must meet state requirements aimed at ensuring the solvency of insurance companies. Provider networks engaged in such arrangements, not surprisingly, disagree.

Currently, the requirements governing such entities vary widely by state. Some states have no requirements at all governing direct contracting arrangements; others—Colorado and Iowa are prominent examples—treat the networks participating in such arrangements as insurers subject to full insurance regulation.

So if you have a problem you think your plan's regulators should be interested in, find out first if your health care coverage is provided through a direct contracting arrangement. If it is, you may have the full protection of your state's insurance department. Or you may have nothing at all.

Who to Call

So far we've only been talking about whether your plan is subject to state regulation, federal regulation, or both. Once you've figured out who is responsible for your plan, you need to find out who to call. This will depend on whether you have private coverage (either through an employer or on your own), Medicare, or Medicaid.

If You Have Private Coverage

You may want to start with the feds because they should be able to tell you whether your problem falls under state or federal jurisdiction. Finding out whom to call is (relatively) easy. The numbers for your region's Labor Department and IRS offices are in every phone book, and most importantly, the agencies have the *same name* in every state, because, of course, they are federal, not state, agencies.

But state regulation of insurance companies—and health care networks such as HMOs that act like insurance companies—is a little more complicated. Remember that there are 50 states—plus the District of Columbia—so there are lots of different ways of organizing—and naming—the same regulatory functions. In some states, three or more agencies may share these functions!

But every state has an insurance department that has a role in licensing and overseeing insurance companies and certain health care networks (check your local phone book for your insurance commissioner's number). Start there. Your state's insurance regulators will tell you what they can handle and will direct you to the agencies that can handle what they can't. See the following page for an example of the type of form your state may ask you to fill out when you file your complaint.

You're on Medicare

You're in luck. Medicare *looooves* to hear from seniors. If you are in a network plan that's not a Medicare HMO, check the back of your Medicare Explanation of Benefits form for how to complain or question a decision by a health care provider or by Medicare itself. Medicare also loves to hear about fraud, so speak up if someone tries to bill you or Medicare for services you have not received.

Your Personal Rx

If you have a problem with your managed care plan that needs to be handled at the state level, your state's insurance commissioner's office is as near to one-stop shopping as you can get. The people there can either handle your problem themselves or identify the people elsewhere in state government that can do so.

```
┌─────────────┐        State Corporation Commission        ┌─────────────┐
│             │              Bureau of Insurance            │             │
│             │           Life and Health Division          │             │
│             │            Post Office Box 1157             │             │
└─────────────┘            Richmond, VA 23218              └─────────────┘
 For Office Use Only                                        For Office Use Only
```

I wish to file a complaint: (please print)

1. My name is: _____ Day Telephone: (_____)_____
                                                                  (Area Code-Number)

2. Mailing Address: _____
                                      (Street/Apt. Number)

   City: _____ State: _____ Zip: _____

3. If you are not the insured or the person on whose behalf this complaint is being filed, please tell us who is and explain your relationship:

   _____

   _____

4. I am complaining against: _____
                              (Name of Insurance Company, Agent or Health Maintenance Organization (HMO))

   _____
                                      (Address, if known)

5. The Insured's policy, Certificate or ID Number is: _____

5. The type of insurance is: ☐ Life   ☐ Health   ☐ Annuity   ☐ Credit

   My Insurance Plan is: ☐ Group   ☐ Individual   ☐ HMO*

*__Note:__ *HMOs are required by law to have internal grievance procedures for their members, and the procedure to follow is explained in your contract of coverage. Before filing a complaint against an HMO, you are urged to take advantage of your HMO's grievance procedure. If your HMO complaint involves quality of care issues, the Bureau of Insurance will forward your complaint to the Virginia Department of Health for a response.*

   The details of my complaint are: (type or print clearly, use other side if needed)

   _____

   _____

   _____

   _____

   _____

   _____

   _____

I am enclosing copies of all correspondence or other papers relating to this matter that may assist the Bureau of Insurance, or the Department of Health, in its evaluation of my complaint. I understand and agree that a copy of this form and any or all of the enclosed information may be provided to the party complained against. I also agree that by signing this form I authorize the Bureau of Insurance, or the Department of Health, to obtain any information required to evaluate my complaint.

   _____   _____
            (Date)   (Signature)

Sample complaint form.

If you're in a Medicare HMO, look in the U.S. government section of your telephone directory for the Medicare listing. There is usually a toll-free number for beneficiary use—that means you.

You're on Medicaid

If you are in a Medicaid managed care plan, your plan is operating under a waiver of standard Medicaid statutes (more on this in Chapter 11). This can be good news for you if your plan is not providing the care you have been promised or believe you are entitled to: Waivers have to be renewed! So if your plan is not delivering for you, the renewal of its waiver could be at risk.

If you have a problem with your plan, first contact your local Department of Social Services (depending on the state, the name of the agency could be different, but it would be the place where you first enrolled in Medicaid). If that office won't or can't help you, contact the state office—it will be in your state capital and may have a toll-free number—or call the Health Care Financing Administration in Washington, D.C. If you are enrolled in a Medicare or Medicaid managed care plan that also accepts other customers, you may also be able to complain to your state insurance commissioner's office, but don't start there.

Caution
If you are enrolled in a Medicare or Medicaid managed care program, *don't* start with your state insurance commissioner if you have a problem. Medicare and Medicaid are largely separate from private insurance programs and are regulated directly by the federal and state governments.

Accreditation

A license means a managed care organization—or doctor or hospital participating in the organization—may legally provide health care. Accreditation is intended to ensure the quality of that care.

An accredited plan meets certain professional standards, which provides the consumer certain safeguards. Accrediting organizations measure whether a plan has structures and systems—such as provider credentialing and utilization management—in place to deliver quality care. Unlike licensure, accreditation is voluntary. However, employers are increasingly requiring that plans they offer either be accredited or be in the process of obtaining accreditation.

Accreditation measures the *process* of delivering health care, not the results. It does not measure differences in patient outcomes. Accreditation also may not reflect patient satisfaction, but only whether processes to measure satisfaction are in place. For example, in a recent survey by *Consumer Reports*, readers gave high marks to some plans with low National Committee on Quality Assurance (NCQA) ratings and low marks to some plans highly rated by the NCQA. (For more on the NCQA, see Chapter 6.) Four organizations currently accredit managed care organizations:

➤ The NCQA

➤ The Joint Commission on the Accreditation of Healthcare Organizations (JCAHO)

➤ The Accreditation Association for Ambulatory Health Care (AAAHC)

➤ The Utilization Review Accreditation Commission (URAC)

House Call

Plans that are denied accreditation may reapply, while those that have previously had full accreditation may lose it. And, depending on the accrediting organization, different levels of accreditation may be possible. So you should be careful that the information you receive is up to date and that you know how to compare information across plans (see Chapter 6 for more on this).

Your Personal Rx
If a health plan isn't licensed, it's probably not accredited, either. Choose a plan that's accredited if you can.

Your Personal Rx
Make sure you try to solve your problem with your plan's member services department or your employer's human resources department before going to regulatory agencies if possible (for more on solving problems with your plan, see Chapter 23). If you have tried to solve the problem, tell the regulatory agencies what you have done and what, if anything, has been the result.

See Appendix B on how to contact these organizations. Some of the organizations accredit all types of plans; the NCQA accredits only HMOs. Each organization looks at somewhat different aspects of the plan in its review.

The NCQA Website contains a list of HMOs—117 as we were writing this book—with accreditation summary reports available (see Appendix B for Websites). Even if your plan is not on the list, it may be accredited, so you should ask. The JCAHO also maintains a Website but asks you to contact their offices to see if your plan or the plan you are considering is accredited. The American Association of Health Plans, an industry group representing managed care organizations, sets voluntary standards that its members are encouraged to meet but does not certify or accredit that those standards are met.

Which Complaints Go Where

Which complaints go to which regulatory agency or level of government depends principally on whether your coverage is paid for through an employer or whether you are buying it on your own.

Complaining About an Employer-Sponsored Plan

If you are in an employer-sponsored plan, and neither the plan's member services department nor your employer's human resources department has been able to help, start with the U.S. Labor Department, the IRS, or both. If your complaint belongs at the state level—perhaps because it deals with a state insurance or licensing issue—either or both of these agencies should be able to tell you.

Complaining About a Plan You Pay for Yourself

If you are paying for your health care coverage on your own—other than COBRA coverage, which comes under the employer coverage heading—federal law does not cancel out state insurance laws in your case. All your state's insurance laws apply to you, and you can sue in state court for whatever the state laws will allow you to. The flip side of that, though, is that neither the Labor Department nor the IRS will step in if you have a problem.

Your plan does have to adhere to certain federal laws, however. These include the Americans with Disabilities Act as well as the Health Insurance Portability and Accountability Act, described in Chapter 7.

The Least You Need to Know

➤ Your plan may have to answer to both federal and state regulators for the rules it sets and how it enforces them. If you don't know whether your problem should be treated at the federal or state level, call the feds first. They should know.

➤ If your health plan is sponsored by your employer, many important state insurance laws and protections may not apply to you. But most health plans or the insurance companies sponsoring them still have to be licensed by the appropriate state agencies.

➤ If your problem needs to be treated at the state level, start with your state insurance commissioner's office. That office has at least part of the responsibility for regulating your health plan and will know who has the rest of the responsibility. The consumer hot line in your state insurance commissioner's office is there to help.

➤ Medicare and Medicaid managed care plans are different from those sponsored by employers or those you buy on your own. If you have a problem, go directly either to Medicare or to your local Department of Social Services.

➤ A license means a plan can operate legally; accreditation is intended to ensure high quality. Make sure any information you get on accreditation is up to date and in a form you can use to compare plans.

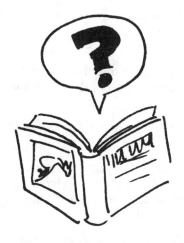

Glossary of Health Care Terms

Arbitration   A dispute resolution process involving a hearing outside a court. The arbitrators, who are supposed to be neutral, hear a complaint and resolve the dispute. That resolution is final and binding on all parties.

Board-certified   A doctor or other health care professional who has passed a test given by their national specialty organization. Board-eligible doctors may be awaiting their exam results or may have completed approved training and may be waiting to take the exams.

Cafeteria plan   An employee benefit plan that allows employees to choose benefits from a number of different options, including pensions and savings, health, other insurance, and time off.

Capitation   A fixed prepayment to a provider to deliver medical services to a certain group, such as all the members of a particular health plan.

Carve-outs   Medical services that are separated from the rest of the arrangements of a managed care plan and contracted for separately.

Case management program   A program that provides comprehensive health care services tailored to the patient's needs. Case managers are usually allowed to provide services not usually covered under the plan, or in settings that may not usually be covered, such as the patient's home, if deviating from the plan's rules meets the patient's needs better.

Certified nurse-midwife   A health care practitioner educated in the two disciplines of nursing and midwifery. That person has graduated from an accredited school of midwifery, acquired national certification, and is licensed to practice in the state.

Certified registered nurse anesthetist   A registered nurse with training and certification in anesthesiology, who may substitute for an anesthesiologist in many surgical procedures.

Chiropractor   A medical professional who treats disease based on the theory that disease is caused by interference with nerve function, and uses manipulation of the joints and the spine to restore normal function.

Chronic condition   A condition that lasts a long time, or recurs frequently, and can be treated but not eradicated.

Clinical trial   An investigation of new methods, materials, or procedures in the treatment of a particular disease or condition. Clinical trials may study ways to prevent, detect, diagnose, control, and treat various diseases, as well as the psychological impact of the diseases and ways to improve the patient's comfort and quality of life.

Coinsurance   The share of the provider's charges, usually a percentage, that the plan member and the plan each pay.

Complementary and alternative medicine   This term covers a broad range of healing philosophies, approaches, and therapies. They can be used alone (often referred to as alternative), in combination, or in addition to conventional therapies (often known as complementary).

Conversion coverage   After employer-sponsored coverage ends, this coverage is purchased directly from your insurance company or managed care plan.

Copayments   Fixed-dollar payments the patient makes per doctor visit or prescription filled. For example, many HMOs and PPOs impose a copayment (sometimes called a "copay") of $5 or $10 for an in-network physician visit.

Covered services   The medically necessary treatments your plan undertakes to pay for, at least in part.

Deductible   The amount of covered expenses an individual must pay before any charges are paid by the medical care plan.

Destination retirement county   A county in which at least 15 percent more people age 65 and older are moving in than are moving out.

Detoxification   The use of medication and other methods under medical supervision to reduce or eliminate the effects of alcohol or substance abuse.

Direct access   Allows you to go to another doctor without having to first go to your primary care doctor (or get a referral) by law. Obstetrics and gynecology are the most common specialties covered by direct access, but others have also gotten under the umbrella.

Discharge planning department   A hospital department that coordinates the follow-up care and other resources a patient leaving the hospital will need to continue recovering at home.

Dual Choice   A POS plan with the option of using an HMO. There is also *triple choice*, dual choice with an addition of a PPO.

Emergency   The sudden onset of a condition or an accidental injury requiring immediate medical or surgical care.

Entry-age rating   An insurance rating system under which your age sets the rate you pay upon entering the plan but does not change as you age. Under attained-age rating, your premium increases every year.

ERISA (Employee Retirement Income Security Act)   A federal law that pre-empts state insurance laws insofar as they apply to private-sector employee benefit plans.

Exclusions   Medical coverages, services, or conditions for which a particular health care plan or policy will not provide or pay.

Exclusive Provider Organization (EPO)   A managed care plan with features of both an HMO and a PPO. Members are only covered for care delivered by network providers. EPOs are generally regulated under state insurance laws.

Extended care facilities   Places that provide skilled nursing care, rehabilitation, and convalescent services to patients requiring less intensive treatment than a hospital provides.

Federal waivers   The legal instruments that allow states to require some or all Medicaid beneficiaries to enroll in managed care plans, or to implement managed care in only part of the state. Waivers can also allow states to test new ways of administering Medicaid plans, including enrolling beneficiaries in plans that serve mostly Medicaid beneficiaries and extending coverage to low-income individuals and families not eligible for "traditional" Medicaid.

Fee-for-service   Method of reimbursement in which doctors bill insurance companies and receive reimbursement for services rendered. A physician or other health care provider bills for each service, with no limits or oversight of the treatment decisions.

Flexible spending account   An account that allows employees to set aside pretax earnings to pay for benefits or expenses that are not paid by their insurance or benefit plans. A flexible spending account may be free-standing or part of a cafeteria plan.

Food and Drug Administration (FDA)   This is the federal agency that evaluates and approves prescription drugs.

Formulary   A list of drugs or classes of drugs preferred by a health care plan for use by its enrollees. In an "open" formulary, the patient does not incur any financial penalties for using nonformulary drugs. In an "incentive-based" formulary, the patient pays a higher copayment for such drugs. In a "closed" formulary, nonformulary drugs are not covered at all.

Gatekeeper   The doctor, usually a primary care doctor, pediatrician, or internist, responsible for overseeing and coordinating all aspects of a patient's care. In an HMO, all referrals, except emergencies, must be preauthorized by the gatekeeper.

Generic substitution   This is the replacement of a prescription drug with another product containing the same active ingredient in the same amount and dosage form, but sold by a different company. All states have laws permitting generic substitution.

Genetic information   Information that concerns genes, gene products, and inherited characteristics of an individual or a family member. Included is information regarding carrier status and information derived from laboratory tests, physical medical examinations, family histories, and direct analysis of genes or chromosomes.

Grievance   A complaint that something that is happening in your health plan is unjust, does not meet the terms of the plan, or causes injury. A grievance is a formal procedure.

Health Care Financing Administration (HCFA)   The federal agency that administers both Medicare and Medicaid (the federal-state program that covers low-income persons and some people in nursing homes).

Health Maintenance Organization (HMO)   A corporate entity (profit or not-for-profit) that provides or arranges for coverage of certain health services for a fixed, prepaid premium.

Health Plan Employer Data Set (HEDIS)   A set of health care quality measure developed by the National Committee for Quality Assurance consisting of statistics on health care delivered by plans, including preventive care and rates for certain surgical procedures.

Home health care   Skilled nursing and related care supplied to a patient at home. Such care may be available only to someone who was previously hospitalized and is recovering without need of hospital care.

Hospice care   Care given to terminally ill patients—generally those with six months or less to live—and emphasizing meeting emotional needs and coping with pain. Care may be given in the patient's home or in a separate facility.

Hospital outpatient department   A facility where a full range of non-urgent medical care is provided under the supervision of a physician.

Indemnity plan   A plan that pays health insurance benefits in the form of cash payments rather than services.

Independent Practice Association (IPA)   An organization of doctors and other medical practices that is formed to negotiate with an HMO to provide medical services.

Integrated delivery system   A health care system that combines health care providers like hospital, doctors, and other medical staff and professionals under one organizational structure to provide a broad base of health care services. They often contract as one entity to several different health plans.

Medicaid   A government program that provides medical assistance for certain low-income individuals and families.

Medically necessary treatments   Those treatments that are appropriate for the diagnosis, care, or treatment of a certain injury or condition.

Medicare   A health insurance program for people over age 65, the disabled, and people with end-stage renal disease who require dialysis or transplantation.

Mid-level health care professionals   Professionals such as nurse practitioners, nurse-midwives, physician assistants, and certified registered nurse-anesthetists that, though they must practice with or under the supervision of a physician, make many patient management decisions on their own.

Nurse practitioner   A registered nurse who has completed an advanced training program in primary health care delivery.

Off-label use   A use that has not been formally approved by the U.S. Food and Drug Administration of a prescription drug that has been approved for other uses.

Osteopathic physician   Doctor with training that places special emphasis on the relationship between the musculoskeletal system and the body's other systems.

Outcomes   Measurement of the impact of the health care system—doctor visits, hospital stays, surgeries—on specific measures of patients' health. Such measures include survival rates and complication rates after various surgeries.

Physician assistant   Works with or under the supervision of a physician to provide diagnostic or therapeutic care. Most are trained in programs granting associate or bachelor's degrees.

Plan administrator   The person or firm designated by your health plan or employer to handle day-to-day details of record-keeping, claims handling, and filing of reports.

Plan participant or beneficiary   An employee or dependent of that employee who is participating, receiving benefits, or eligible to receive benefits from an employee benefit plan.

Point of Service (POS) Managed care plan that allows patients to see doctors not included in the plan for an increased fee. Usually found as part of an HMO.

Portability The ability to carry health coverage from job to job and from group plans to individual coverage.

Pre-existing condition A condition—mental or physical—that began before the plan member became covered under a particular plan.

Preferred Provider Organization (PPO) An arrangement between doctors and others who provide medical services and an insurer to offer services at a discounted rate in exchange for the insurer sending patients their way. It usually has some utilization review.

Primary payor The health care plan that pays its share of covered expenses first, when a consumer has access to two different health plans. The *secondary payor* pays some or all of the amounts left over, even if that amount is less than the secondary plan would otherwise pay.

Provider Whoever provides health care from your health plan. It includes doctors, therapists, nurse-practitioners, and anyone else who provides medical services.

Provider discount Reduced rates that doctors, hospitals, and other health care professionals or facilities agree to accept when they enroll in a health plan's network.

Prudent layperson standard Under this standard, emergency care is covered in a health care plan if the decision to go to the ER was one that an average person with average medical knowledge would make at the time.

Rehabilitation A program designed to change patients' behavior after they are free of acute physical and mental complications from substance or alcohol abuse withdrawal.

Release A current authorization by which you allow specified medical information to be released to a specific person or entity.

Rural areas Towns with fewer than 2,500 people, areas of open country, or counties with a central city (or twin cities) with fewer than 50,000 people. Areas on the outskirts of large cities are generally not considered rural.

Self-insured Describes a plan that pays for medical claims as they arise rather than contract for coverage from an insurer.

Specialty HMOs Organizations similar to HMOs specialize in a particular set of health issues, like dental or mental health.

Telemedicine The use of interactive audio and visual links to enable rural health practitioners to consult in "real time" with specialists in distant medical centers.

Therapeutic effect The way a drug works to cure or heal the condition for which it is prescribed.

Therapeutic substitution   The replacement of a prescribed drug with an entirely different drug of the same pharmacological or therapeutic class. Most state laws are silent on therapeutic substitution.

Urgent care clinic   A facility that provides care for problems that need to be treated outside routine business hours but that are not serious enough to require emergency room care.

Urgent condition   A condition that needs treatment within 24 hours to prevent it from turning into a serious or life-threatening illness.

Utilization review or **utilization management**   The practice in which teams of doctors, nurses, and other health care professionals review the treatment history of patients in order to evaluate the appropriateness of their health care treatment.

Vital signs   A patient's temperature, pulse, and blood pressure.

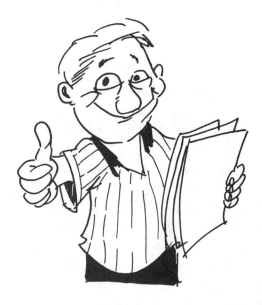

From Print to Plug-In: Health Care Resources

The following is a list of some of the materials we read and used for this book. Some are government publications, some are academic journals, and some are from the magazines and newspapers at your supermarket.

We've also included a list of organizations that can be useful. Some are trade organizations, so their materials also try to make their case. But even these can be useful to you if you can get past the sales pitch.

There is a lot of material out there, piling up every day. And it is *very* accessible. You can also find much of the print material on the Internet and in the library. Almost every trade and professional association, disease group, and government office has a toll-free number. Call the toll-free directory and ask for the group's toll-free number.

We've given a lot of emphasis to Websites (even though we know they can be frustrating) because they can often help shorten your search for the right person to contact or basic information you need. If you don't have Internet access, your local library may be able to help you in your search. Here's a sampling.

Print

Articles and Reports

AIDS Action Foundation. *Medicaid Reform & Managed Care*. Washington, D.C.: AIDS Action Foundation, undated.

American College of Emergency Physicians. *Home Organizer for Medical Emergencies*, Dallas, Texas, 1996.

Annas, George. "Patients' Rights in Managed Care—Exit, Voice, and Choice." *New England Journal of Medicine* (July 1997).

Bodenheimer, R.S., and Kevin Grumbach. "Capitation or Decapitation, Keeping Your Head in Changing Times." *Journal of the American Medical Association*, vol. 276, no. 13 (October 1996): 1025–1031.

"Can HMOs Help Solve the Health-Care Crisis?" *Consumer Reports* 61 (October 1996): 28–35.

DeCarlo, Tessa. "Making Managed Care Work For You." *Glamour* (September 1996): 286–318.

Eisenberg, D. "Advising Patients Who Seek Alternative Medical Therapies." *Annals of Internal Medicine* 127 (1997): 61–69.

Eisenberg, D. et al. "Consumer Information Development and Use." *Health Care Financing Review* 18 (Fall 1996): 15–30.

For the Record: Protecting Electronic Health Information. National Research Council, National Academy Press, 1997.

Goldman, Janlori and Deirdre Mulligan. *Privacy and Health Information Systems: A Guide to Protecting Patient Confidentiality*. The Center for Democracy and Technology, 1996.

Hellinger, Fred J. "The Expanding Scope of State Legislation." *Journal of the American Medical Association* (JAMA), vol. 276, no. 13: 1065–70.

"How Good Is Your Health Plan?" *Consumer Reports* 61 (August 1996): 28–42.

Jewett, Jacquelyn J. and Judith H. Hibbard. "Comprehension of Quality Care Indicators: Differences Among Privately Insured, Publicly Insured, and Uninsured." *Health Care Financing Review* 18 (Fall 1996): 95–110.

Kemper, Donald W. et al. *Kaiser Permanente Healthwise Handbook*. Boise, Idaho: Healthwise, Inc., 1994.

Langreth, Robert. "To Pick the Right HMO, Ask the Right Questions." *Wall Street Journal*, October 28, 1996.

Laurence, Leslie. "Is Managed Care Good for Women's Health?" *Glamour* (August 1996): 202–40.

Long, Stephen H. *Prescription Drug Coverage and the Elderly: Issues and Options*. Washington, D.C.: American Association of Retired Persons, 1994.

"Managed Health Care: Effect on Employers' Cost Difficult to Manage." U.S. General Accounting Office Report, October 1993.

McCormack, Lauren et al. "Medigap Reform Legislation of 1990: Have the Objectives Been Met?" *Health Care Financing Review* 18 (Fall 1996): 157–74.

Pear, Robert. "HMOs Asserting Immunity in Suits Over Malpractice." *New York Times*, November 17, 1996.

Putting HEDIS to Work. Employers' Managed Health Care Association, 1996.

Books

Anders, George. *Health Against Wealth*. Boston: Houghton Mifflin Company, 1996.

Castle Connolly Medical, Ltd. *How to Find the Best Doctors, Hospitals, and HMOs for You and Your Family*. New York: Castle Connolly Medical Ltd., 1995.

Dixon, Barbara. *Good Health for African-American Kids*. New York: Crown Trade Paperbacks, 1996.

Ferguson, Tom. *Health Online*. Reading MA: Addison-Wesley Publishing Company, 1996.

Gray, Bradford H. *The Profit Motive and Patient Care: The Changing Accountability of Doctors and Hospitals*. A Twentieth Century Fund Report, 1991.

Inlander, Charles B. and Ed Weiner. *Take This Book to the Hospital With You: A Consumer Guide to Surviving Your Hospital Stay*. The People's Medical Society, Pantheon Books, 1991.

Kognstvedt, Peter R., ed. *The Managed Health Care Handbook*, third edition. Gaithersburg, MD: Aspen Publishers, 1996.

Lynn, Stephen G. *Medical Emergency! The St. Luke's Roosevelt Hospital Center Book of Emergency Medicine*. New York: Hearst Books, 1996.

Men's Maintenance Manual. Men's Health Magazine, Emmaus, PA, Rodale Press, 1997.

Miller, Marc S., Martha S. Grover, and Philippe Villers. *Health Care Choices in the Washington Area*. Washington, D.C.: Families USA Foundation, 1995. (Titles for other cities also available.)

The Managed Care Information Center. *The Managed Care Yearbook*. Wall Township, NJ: The Managed Care Information Center, 1997.

U.S. Health Care Financing Administration. *Your Medicare Handbook*. Baltimore, MD: Health Care Financing Administration (annual).

Organizations and Websites

The Accreditation Association for Ambulatory Health Care (9933 Lawler Ave., Skokie, IL 60077, tel. 847/676-5411).

The **American Association of Health Plans** (www.aahp.org) is the trade organization for HMOs. They do have consumer materials, and you can check out their bookshelf section on their Website.

If you pick up your phone book, you'll probably see a listing for **American Association of Retired Persons** (AARP). They depend heavily on their local affiliates. They also sponsor meetings on healthcare.

The **American Health Information Management Association** (919 Michigan Ave., Suite 1400, Chicago, IL 60611-1683; www.ahima.org) is the professional association of medical information specialists—those people responsible for your medical records. It has some excellent consumer information.

The **Center for Democracy and Technology** (1634 Eye St., N.W., Suite 1100, Washington, D.C. 20006; www.cdt.org). The center is involved in issues of privacy, electronic recordkeeping, and medical records, among others.

Families USA (1334 G St., N.W., Washington, D.C.20005; www.epn.org/families) is a major player in the health care debate and a source of consumer information as well.

Health Pages (www.thehealthpages.com) is a magazine that offers helpful general information on using managed care. It also provides comparative information on a number of major market areas across the country.

The **March of Dimes** (www.noah.cuny.edu/pregnancy/march_of_dimes/genetics/) is a great source of information as close as your local phone book. Their *Ask Noah* Website is particularly good on prenatal genetic testing and counseling.

The **National Association of Insurance Commissioners** (www.naic.org) has offices in Kansas City, New York, and Washington, D.C. Their Website can give you the name and address of your insurance commissioner and department of health. They also have a help desk.

The **National Committee on Quality Assurance** (2000 L Street, N.W., 20036 Washington, D.C. tel. 800/839-5487; www.ncqa.org) is the private accreditation group for HMOs.

The **National Conference of State Legislatures** (www.ncsl.org) has information about issues such as health and managed care, and laws, regulations, and legislation in the state legislatures.

The **Utilization Review Accreditation Commission** (1130 Connecticut Ave., N.W., Suite 450, Washington, D.C. 20036, tel. 202/296-0120).

Health Care Plan Websites

If you want to check out what your health plan has to say, many of them are also online. You can find the Website address on your plan's newsletters, or you can use one of the Web's many search engines. Some of health plan's Websites provide excellent information, while others are just one step away from a commercial. It's the luck of the draw.

The **California Business Group on Health** has put together a Website (www.healthscope.com) that helps explain your choices, if you are in their area, and provides good data for comparing plans. It is an example of things to come.

The **Center for the Study of Services** (www.consumer.checkbook.org) also has excellent material about comparing hospitals and health plans throughout the country.

Medical Information Websites

Whether you want to check the dailies for the newest health stories or you have questions about an illness, these Websites give you a sampling of what you can find.

If the Websites in the following list don't have the information you're looking for, **Medscape** (www.medscape.com) has links to information on a vast array of subjects, whether you want to read about managed care, mental health, or urology. News services like **Reuters Health** (www.reutershealth.com) can get you up-to-the-minute health news: Check it out if you're an information junkie. And if you want to read some of what your doctor is reading, check out the information in the **New England Journal of Medicine** (www.nejm.org).

American Cancer Society (www.cancer.org)

American College of Sports Medicine (www.acsm.org)

American Diabetes Association (www.diabetes.org)

National Women's Health Network (www.fitnesslink.com/feature/assoc.htm#nwh)

Clinical Trials for Cancer (cancernet.nci.nih.gov/clinical_trials)

Other Clinical Trials (www.centerwatch.com/). CenterWatch provides information on clinical trials in all areas. It als has other information for patients and professionals.

The Centers for Disease Control and Prevention (www.dc.gov)

National Institutes of Health (www.nih.gov)

National Wellness Institute (www.welnessnwi.org)

Index